Managing Brea
in Clinical Prac

Sara Booth • Julie Burkin
Catherine Moffat • Anna Spathis

Managing Breathlessness in Clinical Practice

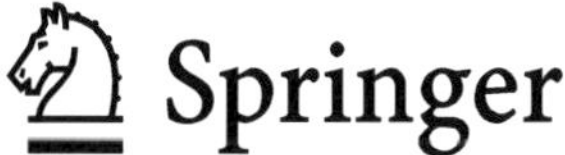

Sara Booth
Department of Palliative Care
Cambridge University Hospitals
NHS Foundation Trust
Cambridge
UK

Catherine Moffat
Department of Palliative Care
Cambridge University Hospitals
NHS Foundation Trust
Cambridge
UK

Julie Burkin
Department of Palliative Care
Cambridge University Hospitals
NHS Foundation Trust
Cambridge
UK

Anna Spathis
Department of Palliative Care
Cambridge University Hospitals
NHS Foundation Trust
Cambridge
UK

ISBN 978-1-4471-4753-4 ISBN 978-1-4471-4754-1 (eBook)
DOI 10.1007/978-1-4471-4754-1
Springer London Heidelberg New York Dordrecht

Springer is part of Springer Science+Business Media (www.springer.com)

This book is dedicated to the patients and their families who suffer with breathlessness throughout the world. We would particularly like to pay tribute to those seen by Cambridge Breathlessness Intervention Service (CBIS) over the years who have participated in research at a difficult time in their own lives and assisted in developing both the service and knowledge that will help other people living with this difficult, intractable symptom.

Sara Booth, Julie Burkin,
Catherine Moffat,
Anna Spathis

Foreword

This book has been written to help clinicians give the best care possible to people suffering from the effects of intractable breathlessness from advanced disease. The word people is used here, rather than patients for several reasons. First, although intractable breathlessness is managed primarily within a clinical, medical system it is important to remember that it is a lived, personal experience affecting all aspects of an individual's life. Many of the most effective interventions for chronic intractable breathlessness include 'lifestyle changes' and therefore any treatment strategy needs to be directed by the person who is both living with the effects of the symptom and who will have to make changes in the way they live to ameliorate it. Secondly, chronic intractable breathlessness affects not only the person who suffers from it but also their immediate friends and family who hear it and see it affecting their relative or friend and who are also limited by its impact on family life.

All this makes for complexity both in assessment and management. In this book the separate elements of these two processes are examined and discussed separately and then a way of integrating them into a management strategy tailored for and lead by the individual patient is outlined. The book is written by members of the Cambridge Breathlessness Intervention Service (CBIS) a service that has been modelled and evaluated using the MRC framework for complex interventions and shown to be effective. CBIS also uses evidence from the growing body of breathlessness research and from other relevant areas. It is a multi-disciplinary team comprising Allied Health Professionals (Julie Burkin and Catherine

Moffat) and a consultant physician (Dr Anna Spathis) backed up by an administrative assistant (Pauline Kleanthous) and with access to consultant psychologist (Dr Nadine Hobro). It is based within a specialist palliative care department in an acute hospital and combines the palliative model of care with a rehabilitative approach. There are few references to specific CBIS practices in the book which is aimed at giving the best care for patients with chronic breathlessness in any setting by any clinician but where relevant direct reference to CBIS is made . What is clear is that even where there is no formal breathlessness service available; helping patients with this difficult and distressing symptom requires a multi-professional, rehabilitative approach where symptom control is addressed with the same fervour as diagnosis and disease management.

Fortunately, in an era where the costs of drugs and other developments in medicine are spiralling and becoming unavailable to many people across the world, and the prevalence of breathlessness is rising, many of the treatments for breathlessness can be used in any setting without elaborate equipment. They do require motivated, empathetic clinicians with the will and knowledge to give the best care. This book is designed to support those clinicians with information and practical help written in an easily accessible form.

The book is organised so that although each chapter refers to other relevant sections, it can be read on its own. There are few references used and these are generally not repeated in the book (so that a greater total number are available for those who want to find out more); each chapter finishes with important key points. It is designed to be carried about to clinic or home, marked, used and worn out. We do hope that you will find something of immediate practical benefit to the breathless patients you see.

Cambridge, UK Sara Booth

Acknowledgements

The authors would like to thank the following people.

Pauline Kleanthous administrative assistant on CBIS since its inception who has done so much to support both the clinical and research work of the service. Malika Harbourn, physiotherapist who has introduced acupuncture to CBIS. Dr Nadine Hobro, consultant psychologist, whose essential work is so valued by her colleagues.

The CBIS evaluation resulted from a collaboration between Sara Booth, Professor Irene Higginson of the Cicely Saunders Institute, Department of Palliative Care and Policy, Kings College London, and Dr Morag Farquhar now of the Institute of Public Health, University of Cambridge.

Earlier clinicians on CBIS, who contributed to the model, Carole Chivertion, Petrea Fagan, Janet Ellis and Megan Forsdyke. Jacquie Adie and Maureen Frostick were also important members of the service when they worked, at different times, as Dr Booth's PA and contributed to the research, strategic and clinical work of CBIS.

Professor Claudia Bausewein, Dr Graeme Rocker and Professor Miriam Johnson have all been close collaborators in developing the research and clinical ideas for breathlessness services.

Contents

Part V An Integrated Strategy

Part I
Introduction

Chapter 1
Breathlessness; the Experience for the Patient, an Approach for the Clinician

It has helped her, which is the important thing … My wife's been, not necessarily sorted, but understanding what she can and can't do better … it takes a lot of stress and worry away from us.

Mrs Brown is now 70 years old. In some ways she feels relieved to have reached this age, she feels so ill during her chest infections that set off an 'exacerbation' of her COPD that she has expected to die several times in the last 10 years. Last winter was particularly bad; she was in hospital six times between October and March, and had to have IV antibiotics and be on non-invasive ventilation (NIV) continuously for 4–5 days, on two occasions. Mrs Brown is sure she is definitely not as active as when that last winter started, she knows she has lost ground physically and now she has to use nocturnal NIV ventilation every night. Mr Brown has started to sleep in the spare room as the machine is so noisy; she has a bell by the bed in case she needs help to get up to go to the lavatory or if she gets frightened. Mind you, if she gets frightened, he does too, and they both feel panicky and usually have a row, which makes them both feel bad.

At least it is May now and she can look forward to better times for a few months, even letting the idea of next winter come into her mind makes her feel apprehensive and it is months away. Trying to stop people visiting if they have a cold, avoiding the surgery, sitting away from people at out-patients who are blowing their noses, wiping down metal door handles at the hospital, feeling worried when items about 'flu appear on the

S. Booth et al., *Managing Breathlessness in Clinical Practice*,
DOI 10.1007/978-1-4471-4754-1_1,

news. The next chest infection could surely kill her. Mrs Brown is determined to enjoy the spring, she will go out when her daughter, Sheila comes over on a Sunday. Sheila's able to help her get into the car, and Mr Brown cannot manage all the oxygen equipment any longer. He gets frightened when she has a breathlessness attack and they come on now with the slightest exertion, even getting out of the car and walking into the pub has to be done in at least three stages and takes 15 min. She hates using the nasal specs in public and being pushed about in a wheelchair but at least it all helps her to get out of the house. It's better to see the grandchildren away from home, where they can run around and make a noise, they tire her out altogether now but she feels so low if she is not up to seeing them. The oldest one has started smoking, she has tried to warn her, 'Look what it's done to me, I know you feel all right now, but it comes on slowly and by the time you're breathless it's too late.' She remembers not believing that smoking could hurt her, but they didn't have as much information then. How she regrets it now.

This week will be a bad week as she has to go up for a hospital appointment and she always feels exhausted for 3 days afterwards, but it is good to see Dr Patel; she feels reassured that he is checking her over and making sure she has the right medication. If only it wasn't so tiring waiting for the ambulance to arrive to take her to hospital and then again in the evening waiting for it to bring her home. She can do so little for herself now, it makes her feel helpless and so vulnerable.

If only there was something she could do to help her breathlessness.

Features of Chronic Breathlessness

Chronic intractable breathlessness is a frightening, disabling symptom affecting every facet of a person's life and of those closest to them. Mrs Brown's story is a typical one and clinicians who care for patients contending with the chronic breathlessness of advanced disease need to be prepared to think about its wide-ranging impact if they are to give patients the most effective treatments. Often the underlying illness will have been maximally treated and yet the breathlessness will persist.

There is more and more evidence confirming that:

1. Breathlessness is a very common symptom for people living with advanced disease of any sort; not only serious cardio-respiratory disease, both malignant and non-malignant in nature, but also, for example, renal and neurological illnesses.
2. Breathlessness is a terrifying symptom to live with, severely limiting the physical capacity of the sufferer. People with chronic breathlessness often experience depression and chronic anxiety.
3. Breathlessness has profound psychosocial effects on the patient and their carer leading to social isolation, loss of employment, huge physical burdens on the spouse or other carer, who has to take over all the 'activities of daily living' that the sufferer can no longer accomplish. Often the carer is elderly and may have an illness themselves.
4. Breathlessness is still easily overlooked in many clinics and specialties, where the primary focus is on disease management, and symptoms are not actively elicited. Many doctors nurses and other clinicians do not ask patients about how breathless they are, because although they are very confident about managing acute breathlessness they are not at all sure how to help someone with chronic breathlessness.
5. As patients become more and more ill, they often become lost to any system of follow-up including primary care, as they become housebound and their carer finds it difficult to help them leave the house. Therefore patients do not benefit from any changes or improvements in medical treatment for their underlying illness, or see those who could give specialist interventions for symptomatic relief of their breathlessness.

Understanding Chronic Intractable Breathlessness

Breathlessness is a complex experience of the mind and the body, rather than a unidimensional event. It has depth in the moment in which it is actually experienced, affected by whatever else is going on for that patient at that instant; and chronicity, accompanying a person through all the events of their life, worsening as their disease increases in severity and improving if the illness can be treated.

The most widely cited definition of breathlessness is that composed by a working party of the American Thoracic Society in 1999, reviewed and not changed, in 2012, where it is defined as,

> … a *subjective experience* of breathing discomfort that consists of *qualitatively distinct sensations* that varies in intensity. The experience derives from interaction among multiple *physiologic, psychological, social, and environmental factors* and may induce secondary physiological and behavioural responses (ATS, 2012).

This comprehensive description encapsulates all the complexity of breathlessness, perhaps the essence of the symptom is best summed up in the phrase 'the uncomfortable awareness of the need to breathe'.

Breathlessness may be a symptom that develops rapidly; this is characteristic of:

- **Primary malignancy**; sometimes the breathlessness that occurs with newly-diagnosed cancer may be completely reversible with systemic anti-cancer treatment. For example a pleural or pericardial effusion may disappear with chemotherapy. If the disease is cured, the breathlessness does not return. Primary lung cancer is rarely cured.
- **Secondary malignancy**; patients may have a period of feeling well when incurable cancer is in remission, this can last months or even years. When the cancer recurs it can progress rapidly and the onset of breathlessness can match this.
- **Some non-malignant lung diseases** such as Interstitial Lung disease (ILD, IPF, fibrosing alveolitis or its variants). The deterioration in the breathlessness can be frightening because it is so fast and because nothing seems to help.

Rapid progression of breathlessness has the following characteristics:

- the patient goes from being a fit, or relatively fit person who can look after themselves, to someone who is unable to walk a few yards, or complete the normal activities of daily living such as talking, washing or dressing themselves without the onset of severe breathlessness.
- The individual who suffers rapidly–progressive breathlessness is often extremely frightened, their world is changing at a speed which prevents them from adjusting; naturally, understandably, the future can seem terrifying at times.
- The relatives and carers of the person with rapidly progressive breathlessness are often very frightened and experience a sense of helplessness. They often feel conflicting emotions about practical arrangements; they need to work to sustain the family income, they want to come to hospital appointments to find out what is going on and if there is anything that can be done, they know that in reality that the patient cannot get there without them. They often feel they need to be in at least three places at once, home, hospital or picking someone or something up. They may find it impossible to understand how their loved one can change so rapidly, they cannot understand why nothing can be done.

Slowly progressive breathlessness is common in:

- **COPD** which progresses over years rather than months; significant irreversible lung damage has been done before the patient experiences any breathlessness. There is no treatment that can currently reverse the lung damage, the disease is progressive if the person does not, for example, stop smoking or if the pathophysiology is untreatable as in alpha1 antitrypsin deficiency. Occasionally for the highly selected individual with a common illness, or for an unusual chronic lung disease, the condition may be treated or improved by a lung transplant or other surgical technique (e.g. bullectomy in some types of COPD) but this is rare.
- **After chemotherapy for malignancy**: Chronic lung disease can follow treatment for malignancy; the underlying malignant disease is cured but the lungs have been

damaged by, for example, chemotherapy or graft versus host disease has developed after transplant therapy.

Characteristics of slowly progressive breathlessness

- The slow progression of the breathlessness allows time for many patients and their families to make psychological and social adjustments to the patient's reduced physical capacity but this is not invariable, or complete.
- Conversely, because the breathlessness has lasted for many years and progressed steadily throughout that time, it has blighted the lives of those individuals living with breathlessness or those who care for them for what can seem like an eternity. Many family events which should have been uncomplicatedly happy, may have been overshadowed by the complex arrangements needed to ensure the patient could actually attend, or spoiled by illness in the run-up to them, or cancelled if the patient was ill.
- Many hours will have been wasted and effort expended in waiting around for out-patients' appointments, collecting repeat prescriptions, dropping in samples of sputum when exacerbations threaten, making travel arrangements which accommodate oxygen cylinders and other bulky equipment.
- The family may have seen the patient or been told the patient is, apparently near death on a number of occasions. It becomes difficult to believe it is going to happen.

Can Breathlessness Be Palliated?

Whilst it is difficult and requires effort to manage breathlessness successfully breathlessness can be improved, although not reversed. Many of the interventions needed are of limited success used alone and need to be part of a complex intervention i.e. one that consists of a number of distinct treatments that can be used concurrently or separately. The extent of incremental improvement possible in the patient will depend on the effort and application of both the clinician(s) caring for that patient and the patient themselves. The carer will also have an influence on how much the patient will improve. This is partly because their own reactions to the patient's breathlessness can reduce or exacerbate the severity of the symptom and because of the encouragement they may be able to give to help the patient persist in using new techniques to manage it. The carer cannot help if they receive no support in contending with the difficulties and limitations the patient's breathlessness imposes on their own life.

> It is possible to reduce the impact of breathlessness without taking away the symptom. A systematic approach addressing the way the patient and carer think feel and behave about the symptom can be very therapeutic. Patients may experience the same level of breathlessness, sometimes more if they are more active, without the previous concomitant levels of distress.

In later chapters the individual interventions outlined below will be described and discussed in detail. In the final chapter, an integrated approach using all the techniques applied as a complex intervention will be presented.

The approach and the interventions used have been derived from the literature, used and evaluated by mixed methods research in the Cambridge Breathlessness Intervention Service (CBIS) over the last 10 years.

Summary of BIS Approach

> **'You understand how I feel, you explain why I feel it and what I can do to help myself.'**
>
> **–Patient's comment on CBIS intervention**

Listen actively to what the patient and family tell you about their experience of living with chronic intractable breathlessness.

Most patients have never had the chance to tell their story about living with breathlessness. They often receive excellent medical care for their underlying disease but it may not be integrated with their goals and priorities or these may not be understood. Not knowing an individual's fears about their illness or its treatment may lead to misunderstandings and seemingly unwarranted fears and anxieties that the clinician cannot comprehend. Patients rarely have the opportunity to describe the impact of the illness on their lives. Often the carer will not have been asked at all about their opinion of how things have changed for them as a family and certainly not their own reactions and the changes they have to make in their own aspirations and lifestyle.

Active listening involves acknowledging what you have heard and repeating it back to the patient and carers to demonstrate that you have understood what you have been told or to give an opportunity for your impression to be corrected. The evidence from the CBIS evaluation has demonstrated how valuable patients and carers find an opportunity to describe what it is like for them to live with breathlessness, for the difficulties that they are facing and have faced and those they have overcome to be acknowledged and understood.

Adopt a positive problem-solving approach

This is central to the way that BIS works and it is research-based. Right from the start of BIS, we were told how much it was appreciated that CBIS clinicians listened to what patients and carers told them, and how encouraging and supportive patients and carers found the recognition of their achievements in living with breathlessness; the focus being on what patients and carers could still do and not solely on what they had lost through illness and living with such a difficult symptom.

Offer the patient a fan and describe in detail how to use it, demonstrating various techniques combined with breathing exercises

The hand-held fan is a cheap, portable, safe piece of equipment that can be of benefit immediately that it is used. It has been an important part of the CBIS treatment strategy since the service was started. The rationale, described in detail in a subsequent chapter, for using the fan to palliate breathlessness is that oro-facial cooling specifically the area of the face sub served by the second and third branches of the trigeminal (fifth cranial) nerve seems to reduce the sensation of breathlessness. In addition giving someone who suffers from a frightening symptom that may come on unpredictably, a tool that they can use to ameliorate the impact of the symptom gives them back a sense of control, of self efficacy that they will otherwise lack. If breathlessness comes on with exertion and using a fan can shorten the inevitable bout of breathlessness, it may also encourage a sufferer to be more active, which will reduce the deconditioning that will exacerbate breathlessness.

Temper sympathy and acceptance of physical limitations, with a rehabilitative approach

The first step is to listen to the patient and their family actively and sympathetically: in other words, listen to what they have been through, acknowledge the emotional pain and the physical and psychological difficulties in their lives, but then work to see how you can help them become more active, do more for themselves, become able to have a greater sense of their own agency and abilities. In other words, it is essential to take a rehabilitative approach, even as a patient approaches the end of life. This does not entail forcing someone to do something of which they are physically incapable, but helping them to do those things which remain within their power. We have reports of patients very successfully using the fan at the end of life, which some might describe as having a placebo effect; it may be the continuance of something the individual can use independently promoting a sense of being able to do something to help themselves.

It may be more constructive to use the word activity rather than exercise and stress that is encompasses social and psychological contact as well as physical activity.

Again it is important for the patient to know from the outset that it is not yet possible to take intractable breathlessness away completely. It is important to make this clear from the beginning of treatment so that the sufferer does not think something has 'gone wrong' when the breathlessness persists. The aim is to enable the patient to be more active and confident with their breathlessness, so reducing its impact.

Adopt an individualised approach

Try as far as you can within your resources to do things the way the patient wants them. It may not always be possible to see patients at home, as CBIS does; we work from an acute hospital and offer a radically different alternative to outpatients. If you work from a hospice, patients may find it helpful to come to you. There may not be enough people on your team to see patients and carers at home all the time; you have to do what you can with the resources available to you. CBIS does find many advantages to doing at least one home visit including being able to fit an exercise/activity regimen to home circumstances. Many elderly breathless people do not go out much at all in the winter; often they are wary not only of the cold and wind which can make breathlessness worse, but also of falling over on ice and getting another complication. Patients, however, may even choose not to be seen at home in a number of circumstances, but if you are asking them to come up and see you, make sure that you make this as easy as possible. There are many reports of patients being totally exhausted by trips up to hospital or other health institutions.

Pay attention to detail

Ensure that the patient chooses, as far as possible, the modes of treatment with which they are most likely to engage and use actively. The non-pharmacological approaches which form the backbone of the CBIS approach require practice and commitment and regular use. The ideas of what will be most acceptable will come out of active listening and if the patient and carer engage with one idea and find it useful they are more likely to then take up other treatment which was initially less attractive.

Offer support to the Carer

This is central to the CBIS approach and is backed by an ever larger evidence base; the carer needs support of their own, in their own right as an individual. The carers' intellectual understanding of and psychological reaction to breathlessness and your suggested management strategy can have a huge influence on the success of the interventions you will recommend.

In addition, the carer needs help with the suffering they are experiencing as a result of the illness of their spouse or relative.

Summary

It is difficult to manage breathlessness, but as we have learned, it is possible to make a real difference to the lives of patients and their families living with the breathlessness of advanced disease and this difference can be transformative.

CBIS uses a *Breathing*, *Thinking*, *Functioning* approach; it can be a useful aide-memoire to check you have carried out a rigorous multifaceted assessment and considered suitable interventions. Let us see what this would be like with Mrs Brown.

1. **Breathing**: **Underlying disease**; Mrs Brown has COPD and sees Dr Patel every 6 months; Mr Brown says little at the consultations and is frustrated that she does not tell Dr Patel how much worse she is at home now, so much worse that she is not using her inhalers properly and in fact often does not use them at all until an exacerbation threatens. Then she is usually too breathless to manage them. Mrs Brown often does not use the antibiotics she has been given to start in the early stages of an infection. You decide to talk to Dr Patel yourself, with the Mrs Brown's permission, to let him know a fuller picture of what is going on. He is very concerned that Mrs Brown is getting much weaker and may not survive another winter; she needs to use her medication properly. He asks you to see if Mrs Brown will allow the respiratory nurses into her home, something she has refused up until then. You also talk to the GP; he decides that the extra vigilance offered by Mrs Brown being on the Gold Standards Framework Practice Register (highlighting patients who may die within the next year) will be helpful. You discuss breathing exercises, helpful positions to reduce breathlessness and energy conservation and explain about and give her a hand-held fan. You talk to Mrs Brown about using morphine, which you think will be useful in the mix with these other treatments.

2. **Thinking**: **Mr and Mrs Brown** have never really talked together about the COPD and the way it has affected their lives. Whilst you do not set this up as a formal conversation it flows naturally from your detailed assessment visit and subsequent home visit and then telephone conversations. It brings them to a new understanding of what each of them is facing and why they sometimes seem to react, in the other's eyes, unhelpfully at times of crisis. It reduces their sense of isolation. Your detailed discussion and education about the nature of breathlessness, how it can be precipitated and exacerbated assuages a number of fears they have been unable to discuss with each other and which have, at times, caused unbearable, private anxiety. You make an action plan with them together and record their goals of care and the ways you will help them work towards them. You will review these with them on every visit. On your second visit you suggest that Mrs Brown might benefit from going to the hospice day therapy centre, where she can have some gentle rehabilitation. It will give Mr Brown a 'day off' to go to his bowls club where he has many friends, missing it has caused him deep resentment which he has been unable to express. He does not need to now, he can go. Over time, the reduction in anxiety and the changed reactions they both have to episodes of breathlessness mean that these are shorter and less frequent. Mrs Brown is more willing to use the inhalers and start early antibiotics now she has a greater understanding of why she is taking them. She finds the respiratory nurse kind and helpful and has made a good link with the hospice by the time you discharge her from your care after your fourth visit.
3. **Functioning**. **Mrs Brown** is delighted to be able to walk further and faster after some rehabilitation at home and the hospice. She finds the fan and the breathing exercises both helpful and reassuring and is surprised to find how much stronger and how much improved her balance is with more walking. It pleases her to be able to get out of the chair on her own and use the rollator to walk about independently. Mr Brown feels less exhausted as he is less worried and happier because he has some relaxed life of

his own. After Mrs Brown's period of attendance at the hospice ends, a carer comes to her home so that Mr Brown can continue to go out at least once a week for a few hours. Again you review the action plan and help the Browns decided new ways of facing up to the limitations and fears that winter brings.

The *Breathing, Thinking Functioning* approach will be different in emphasis with someone whose breathlessness is relentlessly progressive but the principles are the same and managing the breathlessness that follows both trajectories will be discussed in detail in the chapters that follow.

Key Points

- Breathlessness is a complex experience of the mind and body and the clinician needs to use active listening to understand the patient's and carer's needs
- A rehabilitative approach based on palliative care principles is needed to help the symptom
- Non-pharmacological, procentral interventions can be classified by their main mode of action i.e. helping *breathing, thinking and functioning*
- Carers need support and help for themselves
- Breathlessness may progress rapidly (over days or weeks) or more steadily (over months or years) and this has implications for management.
- Pharmacological therapy is needed when patients have severe intractable breathlessness or at the end of life.

Further Reading

Spathis A, Davies HE, Booth S. Respiratory disease; from advanced disease to bereavement. Oxford: OUP; 2011.

Booth S, Moffat C, Farquhar M, Higginson IJ, Burkin J. Developing a breathlessness intervention service for patients with palliative and supportive care needs, irrespective of diagnosis. J Palliat Care. 2011; 27(1):28–36.

Booth S, Dudgeon D. Dyspnoea in advanced disease: a guide to clinical management. Oxford: OUP; 2005.

Booth S, Moffat C, Burkin J. The BIS manual. Cambridge: Cambridge University Hospitals NHS Foundation Trust; 2012.

Williams S. Chronic respiratory illness. The experience of illness series. Routledge: Chapman & Hall; 1993.

Parshall MB, Schwartzsein RM, Adams L, et al. On behalf of the ATS Committee on Dyspnea. Am J Respir Crit Care Med. 2012;185(4): 435–52.

Gysels MH, Higginson IJ. The lived experience of breathlessness and its implications for care: a qualitative comparison in cancer, COPD, heart failure and MND. BMC Palliative Care. 2011;10:15.

Chapter 2
The Genesis and Assessment of Breathlessness

Introduction

The successful management of any symptom requires an understanding of its genesis. Breathlessness is no exception, and an appreciation of the underlying mechanisms can help direct both effective assessment and treatment. Unlike other symptoms, however, the aetiology of breathlessness is particularly complex, and this occurs for a number of reasons.

Respiration is the only body system vital for survival that is under both volitional and automatic control. There is no advantage in other major organs, for example cardiac or renal function, being under conscious influence. Breathing, however, needs to be controlled precisely when undertaking activities, such as swallowing, speaking or swimming. This means that the neural circuitry must involve higher cortical pathways. The perception of breathlessness is a complicated process that is, as yet, not fully understood.

Further complexity occurs at a clinical level. A vast number of pathological processes can have an impact on respiratory function and cause breathlessness. Diseases of the lung parenchyma and chest wall, neuromuscular and cardiac pathology, as well as a myriad of metabolic conditions, can all influence respiration.

The acute and distressing sense of breathlessness is very useful when there is an immediate threat to survival, such as suffocation or inhalation of a noxious substance. A homeostatic

S. Booth et al., *Managing Breathlessness in Clinical Practice*,
DOI 10.1007/978-1-4471-4754-1_2,

threat needs to generate a rapid emotional response, such as terror, that leads in turn to an adaptive behaviour, such as increasing respiratory effort and running away. However, once the symptom becomes chronic, its perception is less helpful and, indeed, can cause maladaptive emotions and behaviours that actually perpetuate the breathlessness.

Pathophysiological and clinical models have been developed in an attempt to explain these complex processes. This chapter sets out two such models, and outlines how an understanding of these mechanisms can closely guide symptom assessment and management.

Models for Understanding the Genesis of Breathlessness

Pathophysiological Model (Parshall et al. 2012)

The mostly widely accepted theory underpinning the perception of breathlessness is the 'mismatch' theory.

> Breathlessness is experienced when there is mismatch between the demand for ventilation and feedback on actual ventilation. It occurs when ventilatory demand increases or the mechanical process of ventilation is impaired.

The demand for ventilation generates central respiratory motor activity that drives respiration. It is thought that a copy of this efferent information is sent centrally allowing the brain to predict the sensory feedback that should occur. This 'corollary discharge' is compared with the peripheral afferent signals that actually arise, and any mismatch between the two leads to the feeling of breathlessness. This integration appears to occur in the limbic-related cortex, in particular the anterior

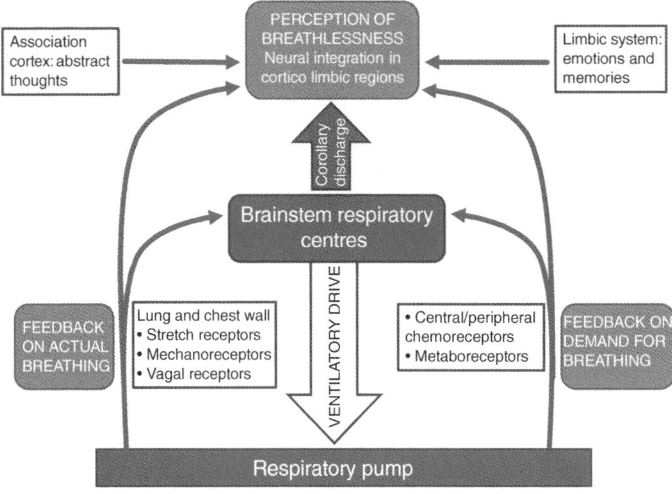

FIGURE 2.1 Pathophysiology of breathlessness (Adapted from Moosavi et al. 2011)

insular region (Schon et al. 2008). This deep inner layer of the brain cortex is involved in awareness of homeostatic threats, and generates emotional and behavioural responses. It can be thought of as an 'internal alarm centre', and appears to play a key role in the genesis of breathlessness. This model is represented schematically in Fig. 2.1.

Although complex and theoretical, there are a number of clinically relevant implications of this model:

- The large number of afferent inputs into the perception of breathlessness leads to a broad range of potential ways of modulating the symptom.
- The close relationship with parts of the brain involved in emotions and thoughts can help clinicians and patients understand the importance of psychological influences on the perception of breathlessness.
- It gives a potential explanation for how other unpleasant sensations, such as pain, extreme heat or negative emotions, can influence breathlessness, as all such threats are perceived in a similar area of the brain.

Mr James: Part A

Mr James had to retire early from his work in the building industry as his health was deteriorating. He knew he had COPD, and his breathing was becoming a real problem, even walking about slowly. He also had bad hip, knee and back pain from arthritis, and had been told that he could not have surgery because of his poor chest. Over the last year he had become completely house bound, and was afraid to leave the house even for medical appointments. His GP told him he was agoraphobic, and arranged for him to see the local mental health services, as well as referring him to you for breathlessness management.

At the first meeting, Mr James expresses his anger about being 'thought of as a loony'. He explains that he is terrified of having a panic when out of the house. This has happened on two occasions; he was terrified and thought he was dying. On detailed questioning he identifies that his breathing is worst on the days when his arthritis is really playing up. His wife says that he sometimes 'shouts out' in pain when he first tries to move after sitting for a while.

You explain to Mr and Mrs James that the part of the brain that feels the breathlessness also deals with other unpleasant feelings like pain. This area is like an 'internal alarm' to the body, and automatically leads to a number of feelings (like fear) and behaviours (like staying still to try to avoid the breathing or pain problems). When you state that it is 'all part of the hardwiring of the brain', and a completely normal response to what is happening, he is visibly relieved and becomes briefly tearful.

Case continued in part B on page…

Breathing, Thinking, Functioning (BTF) Perpetuation Model

This model is the clinical key to the successful management of breathlessness. It both gives an explanation for the perpetuation of the symptom, and leads directly to potential ways of managing it.

In evolutionary terms, there is a clear survival advantage for the perception of a threat to lead to an immediate negative emotion. This in turn motivates behavioural changes to avoid the danger. Once the threat becomes chronic, however, these emotions and behaviours are no longer helpful. Indeed, they can become maladaptive and inadvertently perpetuate the problem.

In chapter 1, the three facets of breathlessness management were introduced: 'breathing', 'thinking' and 'functioning' (or BTF). In each of these, specific unhelpful emotions or behaviours develop. These then lead to three inter-related vicious cycles that prolong and worsen the symptom (Fig. 2.2).

1. **Breathing vicious cycle**

   Patients who are breathless often develop an inefficient breathing pattern. They perceive they need to take big breaths in, 'to get more air', and usually imagine the air coming into the upper part of their chest. Ask any child to take a big breath in, and it usually involves upper chest movement with hunched shoulders. Patients tend to pant, with a small tidal volume shunting air within the respiratory dead space. Accessory muscles of respiration are used in an attempt to pull air into the upper chest. This all greatly increases the work of breathing and reduces its efficiency. Breathlessness worsens and the vicious cycle has developed.

   In patients with air flow obstruction, the situation is compounded by the fact that at increased respiratory rates,

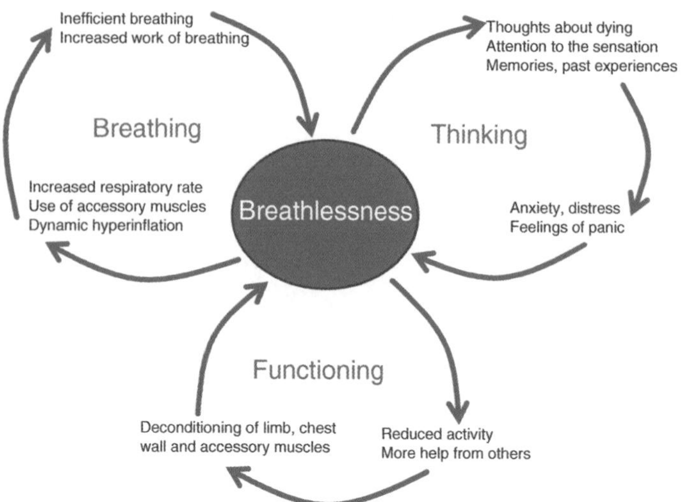

FIGURE 2.2 Perpetuation of breathlessness by vicious cycles

there is insufficient time for the lungs to empty. The next inspiration is initiated before the lungs have deflated fully. 'Breath stacking' occurs, leading to dynamic hyperinflation. This exerts a restrictive mechanical disadvantage on the respiratory muscles; inhalation is hindered by the chest already being over-expanded. Breathing becomes inefficient and the work involved considerable. Furthermore, there is greater reliance on tachypnoea to increase ventilation, reducing further the time for the lungs to empty and compounding the hyperinflation.

2. **Thinking vicious cycle**
As is clear from the pathophysiological model above, breathlessness almost invariably leads to feelings of anxiety or distress. The corticolimbic areas of the brain involved in the perception of breathlessness also deal with the processing of emotion and attention. Heightened anxiety and increased awareness will directly increase the perception of the symptom. This well-recognised vicious cycle can lead to panic, and almost all breathless patients have, at some point, experienced this.

Furthermore, anxiety causes muscle tension, which increases the work of breathing. It also increases the respiratory rate, and can give a sense of needing to gasp or take big breaths in, so contributing further to the breathing vicious cycle described above.

3. **Functioning vicious cycle**

   Breathlessness is an unpleasant sensation. It is natural, therefore, to try to avoid having to experience it, and patients tend to reduce their activity. However, this leads to muscle deconditioning, both of limb muscles and those involved in respiration. Deconditioned muscles are weaker and use oxygen less efficiently, both of which increase the demand on the respiratory system and therefore increase the breathlessness. Patients easily understand this classic 'deconditioning cycle', as it is obvious that people who are less 'fit' become more breathless on exertion.

   Family members and carers unwittingly compound the situation. They try to help by undertaking activities that the patient might otherwise have done. Patients and their carers are usually surprised when they realise that the understandable reduction in activity is actually worsening the situation. However, it can be motivating to know that putting up with the moderate breathlessness caused by increased activity can actually improve the symptom over the longer term and this can contribute to patient engagement in self-management.

This model is of clinical importance for a number of reasons:

- It helps patients, carers and professionals understand why a symptom may be continuing or worsening, when this does not appear to fit with the trajectory of the underlying disease.
- It can guide professionals into understanding which facet(s) of breathlessness management, 'breathing', 'thinking' or functioning', would be the most helpful to focus on.
- Appreciation of the components of the predominant vicious cycle can give specific ideas for symptom management.

Mr James: Part B **continued from page...**

As a healthcare professional, you are now developing an understanding of Mr James' breathlessness. The 'thinking' vicious circle is clearly occurring; he has experienced episodes of panic and has become anxious to the point of not leaving the house. It is also obvious that the 'functioning' vicious circle is a problem. Many factors are contributing to his decreased activity and deconditioning, including severe pain on movement, breathlessness and his inability to leave home.

You explain to Mr and Mrs James that the normal feelings and behaviours that happen in response to breathlessness are not always helpful, and can sometimes lead to vicious circles. Mr and Mrs James listen carefully as you explain the two vicious circles, engaged by the simplicity and logic of the argument. Mr James becomes increasingly animated explaining that he knew that, if he could just move a bit more, things would improve. Deep down he was aware that he was getting really frightened, and was behaving in a way that was so different from the adventurous life he used to lead. He had never even thought of being frightened, harnessed to scaffolding over the years in his building job.

But then his face falls. How will he ever get more active, when the breathlessness is frightening and his pain so severe?

Case continued in part C on page...

Assessment of Breathlessness

Breathlessness, like pain, can only by perceived by the person experiencing it. Adequate assessment relies on self-report. Giving patients the opportunity to tell their story in detail, can be of therapeutic value in itself.

The purpose of a clinical assessment is to understand the causes and consequences of the symptom in a particular patient, so that is can be managed effectively. More specifically, the objectives are to:

- Understand the disease process(es) that underlie the symptom (airway obstruction, pleural effusions, anaemia and so on) allowing potentially reversible pathology to be treated.
- Appreciate which of the 'breathing, thinking, functioning' vicious cycles predominate in perpetuating or worsening the patient's breathlessness, so allowing the management to be focused accordingly.
- Understand the expectations and priorities of the patient and their family, so that expectations can be influenced and consistent goals agreed.
- Quantify the experience of the symptom and its impact, so that any response to intervention can be ascertained.

Almost all of the assessment can be done by taking a careful history. It is ideal if this involves both the patient and key family members. Medical examination and/or investigations can contribute to understanding the underlying disease pathology. The following areas of discussion should be included:

1. Look for reversible causes

    - Establish the speed of onset and temporal pattern of the breathlessness. An acute deterioration may suggest a potentially reversible cause, such as a chest infection.
    - Ask about associated symptoms, for example, sputum production, fever, orthopnoea, syncope, palpitations, weight loss.

2. Breathing

    - Find out what factors precipitate and relieve the breathlessness, including whether the symptom is influenced by body position, type of exertion, room temperature and specific medication.

- It can be interesting to note the words patients use to describe the sensation. 'Air hunger' is associated with increased respiratory drive or dynamic hyperinflation, and appears to be particularly distressing. 'Effort' or 'work' can suggest muscle weakness or fatigue, 'suffocation' can characterise panic attacks, and 'tightness' may suggest bronchospasm.

3. Thinking

   - Ask about patients' understanding of both the causes and consequences of their symptoms and underlying disease. Specifically, some patients feel that the breathlessness is, in itself, causing damage to their body.
   - Find out about their emotional reaction, in terms of anxiety, mood and feelings of panic.

4. Functioning

   - Establish the previous and current levels of activity in some detail, both in and out of their home. Specific questions, such as exercise tolerance walking slowly on the flat, can be helpful.
   - Try to understand social limitations imposed by the symptom, in terms of altered roles, loss of friendships, ability to go shopping etc.
   - Find out if equipment is being used or is needed, such as a frame, kitchen trolley etc.
   - Consider the role of the carer, in terms of additional responsibilities in and out of the home.

5. Expectations and priorities

   - It is helpful to find out patient's expectations in terms of how their problems may change over time. Try also to ascertain their expectations in relation to how a healthcare professional may be able to help.
   - Find out about the patient's priorities. For one patient, being able to walk the dog again may be a priority, whereas for other patients it may be to be able to sleep well at night, or to know that they can abort a panic attack if it arose again.

6. Existing coping strategies

    - All patients will have discovered ways of trying to manage their symptom, even if not apparently coping well. It is enormously revealing to find out what how they have adapted, and the strategies they already use to manage their condition. This may include using medication.
    - Ask specifically about what they do when they are feeling particularly breathless to try to help the symptom settle quickly.

7. Outcome measures

    - Clinical outcome measures are useful both in terms of contributing to understanding the patient's experience, and by allowing the impact of the intervention to be quantified.
    - It is worth using only a small number of simple measures, to reduce the burden on the patient. A numerical rating scale from 0 to 10 is usually easiest for a patient to understand.
    - Measuring the ability of a patient to cope with the breathlessness is often more useful than measuring the severity of the symptom. A patient who is self-managing their symptoms effectively, may be more active and therefore no less breathless.

- How breathless are you these days on a scale of 0–10, where 0 is not breathlessness and 10 is the worst breathlessness you can imagine?
- How anxious are you these days on a scale of 0–10, where 0 is not anxious at all and 10 is the worst anxiety you can imagine?
- How confident are you in managing your breathlessness on a scale of 0–10, where 0 is not confident at all and 10 is extremely confident?
- Since we first met, has your activity level reduced/stayed the same/increased?

Patients' expectations and priorities are particularly important to establish. It may be unrealistic to expect the breathlessness to resolve, whereas it would be entirely reasonable to aim to cope better, feel in control and know what to do when acutely breathless.

The First Assessment: Practical Tips

Some patients find that talking about breathlessness actually makes their breathing feel worse. Usually this manifests as a patient not engaging; occasionally a patient may shut down the conversation. It is important to be aware of this, and in such patients it may be more helpful to focus initially on the value of the fan and relaxation techniques.

A full assessment can take at least an hour, sometimes more. Breathless patients are often fatigued, and may find such a lengthy conversation too exhausting. It is worth therefore considering the assessment and management priorities during the first consultation. The assessment itself may extend over a couple of meetings, running concurrently with management advice.

Particularly when time or patient energy is limited, the following are usually considered as priorities in the first patient meeting:

- Check there is no potentially reversible pathology, such as a chest infection, or a pleural effusion, or other reversible contributor, like pain.
- Identify the patient's own ways of managing the breathlessness. If you are explicit in praising these, it can boost patients' confidence and engagement in self management. Enhancing patients' sense of their own resilience and ability to problem solve is an important professional role.

- Manage patient expectations, and explain that improvement involves small, incremental steps over many weeks. It is an active process, which requires engagement and practice.
- Decide which one or two of the 'breathing', 'thinking' or 'functioning' vicious cycles is the greatest problem and use this to focus the initial management.
- Think about 'quick wins', one or two particularly pertinent or helpful ideas which will help engage the patient in persisting with other breathlessness management techniques. Examples include explaining and using the fan (page 43), developing a short action plan (page 108) or practising the recovery breathing technique (page 100)

Mr James: Part C continued from page…
It is clear from your assessment so far that Mr James has become deconditioned from inactivity resulting from his breathlessness, joint pain, and fear about leaving his house. There is so much you could focus on and discuss, but you can already see that he is getting tired and possibly slightly anxious.

You start by noting positively his considerable insight, including his determination to keep walking within his home, despite his severe arthritic pain. Without this, his condition would be even worse. You can see that his expectations are low, and explain that you believe he will be able to make progress over a number of weeks, but it will involve persistence and patience.

You decide to focus on the 'thinking vicious cycle during this first consultation. He now understands how panic develops and the importance of finding ways to relax and manage his anxiety. You explicitly address his misconception that he might die during a panic attack (very near the end of life 'waste gases' build up and make people feel calm and drowsy, not panicky), describe the recovery breathing technique (page…) and agree a four point action plan' that he can use if he feels frightened.

You end the consultation by leaving him a CD with the narrative of a short relaxation technique. His wife jokes that she 'needs it too', and they agree to listen and practice the technique together each evening.

Your final step is to explain that you will speak with Mr James' GP to discuss ways of improving his pain management. Pain control may benefit him both by reducing his perception of the breathlessness, and also by facilitating activity. Slowly building up his activity will be an essential part of working on the 'deconditioning vicious cycle', the focus of your next consultation...

Key Points

- Although the genesis of breathlessness is multifactorial and poorly understood, the complexity does usefully allow there to be multiple potential approaches to symptom management.
- Patients, carers and clinicians need to understand the extent to which thoughts and emotions impact on the experience of breathlessness.
- The concept of 'breathing', 'thinking' and 'functioning' vicious cycles helps patients and clinicians understand how the breathlessness is perpetuated, and can usefully guide symptom management.

References

Moosavi S, Booth S. The genesis of breathlessness. In: Cambridge breathlessness intervention service treatment manual. Cambridge: Cambridge University Hospitals NHS Foundation Trust; 2011.

Parshall M, Schwartzstein R, Adams L, et al. An official American thoracic society statement: update on the mechanisms, assessment and management of dypsnoea. Am J Respir Crit Care Med. 2012;185(4):435–52.

Schon D, Rosenkranz M, Regelsberger J, et al. Reduced perception of dyspnoea and pain after right insular cortex lesion. Am J Respir Crit Care Med. 2008;178:1173–9.

Part II
Non-pharmacological Interventions – Breathing

Chapter 3
Fan and Oxygen Therapy

Introduction

Breathless patients seem to have an intuitive sense that they need 'more air'. Patients typically seek fresh, moving air, for example by keeping hospital bed curtains open, opening windows and using a fan. As oxygen is the vital constituent of inhaled air, it is not surprising that people equally expect supplemental oxygen to be helpful. The majority of patients and healthcare professionals, including respiratory and palliative care staff, believe that breathless patients benefit from oxygen therapy. Administration of oxygen is an automatic treatment for breathless patients admitted to hospital, and a significant proportion of those with incurable underlying respiratory disease are then prescribed oxygen for use at home.

Some of the dangers of oxygen therapy have long been understood, including the risks of hypercapnic respiratory failure and oxygen toxicity. However, only in recent years has there been an understanding of the need to reduce emergency oxygen administration, with an emerging body of evidence revealing worse outcomes in many patients receiving oxygen. Non-hypoxaemic stroke patients, for example, randomised to oxygen therapy have a higher mortality, and neonates resuscitated with room air appear to do better than those given oxygen. Recent guidance for emergency oxygen

S. Booth et al., *Managing Breathlessness in Clinical Practice*,
DOI 10.1007/978-1-4471-4754-1_3,

use recommends prescribing according to a target saturation range, rather than a flow rate or concentration.

> The target saturation range is 94–98 % for most acutely ill patients and 88–92 % for those at risk of hypercapnic respiratory failure.

Homeostasis is a complex and effective process. Hypoxia leads to a reflex constriction of pulmonary vessels, to reduce ventilation perfusion (VQ) mismatch, and reflex dilatation of cardiac, cerebral and systemic vessels increases oxygen delivery to the tissues. Patients acclimatise to chronic hypoxaemia, and patients with chronic cardiorespiratory disease can, like mountaineers, tolerate low oxygen saturations, often well below 70 %. It is, therefore, unsurprising that hindering normal homeostatic mechanisms with supplemental oxygen can be harmful. Oxygen therapy can worsen VQ mismatch, as well as causing cerebral and cardiac vasoconstriction, reduction in cardiac output, absorption atelectasis and an increase in toxic free radicals.

In this context, one would expect the widespread use of oxygen for palliation of breathlessness to be supported by evidence of benefits outweighing harms. Does this evidence exist? This chapter seeks to outline research evidence both for the use of oxygen and of air, and gives detailed guidance to inform clinical practice.

Oxygen Therapy

Evidence Base

Booth et al. published a seminal paper in 1996, which showed that inhalation of both cylinder oxygen and cylinder air significantly improved breathlessness in hospice cancer patients (Booth et al. 1996). Importantly, there was no difference between the two gases; both oxygen and air led to symptom palliation. A large number of single assessment and pragmatic longer-term studies have since attempted to evaluate the role of oxygen in breathlessness management, and the evidence is summarised in the box below.

Research Evidence

Oxygen can be delivered as long-term oxygen therapy (LTOT) where oxygen is inhaled for 15 or more hours out of every 24 h; as short-burst oxygen therapy (SBOT) with intermittent use before or after exertion; and as ambulatory oxygen therapy given using small cylinders during exertion.

LTOT

In COPD patients with severe hypoxaemia (PaO_2<7.3), there is clear evidence that LTOT increases survival, improves quality of life and relieves breathlessness. In non-hypoxaemic patients, a recent systematic review has revealed a small reduction in breathlessness (equating to 0.9 points in a 0–10 numerical rating scale) of borderline clinical significance (Uronis et al. 2011). Subgroup analysis showed the benefit occurred in LTOT and not SBOT trials. However, this review did not include data from a subsequent RCT which revealed no difference between oxygen and air received for >15 h/day over a 7 day period in a mixed group of predominantly COPD patients (Abernethy et al. 2010). There have been no trials evaluating the use of LTOT in cancer patients.

SBOT and ambulatory oxygen therapy

In non-hypoxaemic COPD patients, as described above, a systematic review has shown no benefit from SBOT. A subsequent RCT in the same patient group also failed to demonstrate benefit from ambulatory oxygen (Moore et al. 2011). In a systematic review of non- or mildly hypoxaemic cancer patients receiving either SBOT or ambulatory oxygen therapy oxygen did not palliate breathlessness (Uronis et al. 2008). In this review, the single positive trial out of the five included studies was the one with the most hypoxaemic patients (all participants $SaO_2 < 90\ \%$).

Although there is little evidence for oxygen improving breathlessness across study populations, within each trial a number of patients did benefit from oxygen.

- The response to oxygen, importantly, does not appear to correlate with the degree of hypoxaemia, degree of desaturation on exercise, or any test of lung function.
- The response is extremely variable between individuals, although more reproducible at an individual level. (Spathis and Booth 2008)

Potential Mechanisms

A number of possible mechanisms of action for oxygen have been proposed of which the most important are as follows:

- *Reversal of hypoxaemia.* Hypoxaemia is a potent stimulus of respiratory drive, which is believed to result in breathlessness by increasing the mismatch between demand for ventilation and feedback on actual ventilation (see page 18) Oxygen therapy prevents this process from occurring.
- *Reduction in blood lactate levels*. Reduction in oxygenation of muscle leads to lactic acid production. This increases ventilatory demand, in an attempt to compensate for the metabolic acidosis. Supplemental oxygen will reduce lactic acid formation. This mechanism could increase the ability to recondition by exercise training, although this may be limited by the fact that there is some evidence that lactic acid production can enhance the training effects on muscle.
- *Reduction in dynamic hyperinflation.* Lung hyperinflation occurs when there is incomplete lung emptying in

obstructive airways disease (see page 94). The functional restriction in inhalation puts greater reliance on tachypnoea to increase ventilation. However, tachypnoea gives less time for full exhalation, leading to a vicious cycle. It is believed oxygen breaks this cycle by reducing the demand for ventilation and therefore the respiratory rate.

- *Stimulation of facial and nasopharyngeal receptors.* Receptors stimulated by a cool flow of gas project afferent information that reduces the perception of dyspnoea; local anaesthesia in this region has been shown to increase breathlessness (Liss and Grant 1988). Oxygen may work simply by providing a flow of a cool gas, and this may explain why studies have shown benefit from both cylinder oxygen and cylinder air.
- *Placebo effect.* The widely held view that oxygen should reduce breathlessness may in itself alter central processing of the sensation through a placebo effect.

The range of potential mechanisms both involved in the genesis of breathlessness (see page 17) and explaining the effect of oxygen (above) may explain why, for individual patients, benefit from oxygen does not appear to correlate with the degree of hypoxaemia. Oxygen in a non-hypoxaemic patient, for example, may help breathlessness by reducing dynamic hyperinflation. Conversely, the breathlessness of a hypoxaemic patient may relate to afferent information from lung or chest wall receptors that is not influenced by reversal of hypoxaemia.

Clinical Guideline for Use of Non-emergency Supplemental Oxygen

This guidance provides a pragmatic approach, based on a combination of current evidence and expert opinion. Although the evidence points to a lack of benefit for oxygen (other than LTOT in hypoxaemic COPD patients), palliation of breathlessness does occur in a few patients. The only way to decide whether or not to prescribe oxygen for a particular patient is to undertake an individual clinical assessment.

An **individual clinical assessment** involves measuring breathlessness severity both with and without supplemental oxygen. This can range in rigour from a formal 'N=1 randomised controlled trial' to a simple explanation about the lack of evidence for oxygen therapy and asking patients to assess critically whether or not they feel oxygen is helping them. In practice, a pragmatic compromise involves selecting a specific activity within a patient's home (such as climbing the stairs), and asking the patient to keep a diary quantifying breathlessness on a 0–10 numerical rating scale after undertaking this activity, both with and without oxygen.

- Oxygen therapy is not appropriate in patients with SpO_2>92 %.
- LTOT should be provided only to severely hypoxaemic COPD patients with a PaO_2<7.3 kPa. This is a lifetime commitment to use oxygen for over 15 h per day. In severely hypoxaemic cancer patients, LTOT can be considered, although the use is not evidence based. LTOT is best supplied by an oxygen concentrator and delivered via nasal cannulae, with access to ambulatory oxygen.
- Ambulatory oxygen alone can be considered in less hypoxaemic patients with exercise desaturation, specifically when the SpO_2 falls by >4 % to below 90 % during exercise. Its effectiveness must still be checked by recording the distance a patient can walk and the dyspnoea severity (with 0–10 numerical rating scale) both with and without oxygen. Lightweight portable cylinders are available.
- Use of SBOT is *not* recommended unless intermittent hypoxia is suspected and the breathlessness has not been relieved by any other treatment. In this case, an individual clinical assessment is warranted. In practice the majority of patients benefit more from use of handheld fan than from SBOT (see below).

- When oxygen is prescribed, as with emergency oxygen prescription, a flow rate should be used that keeps the SpO_2 within a target range: 88–92 % for those at risk of hypercapnaeic respiratory failure and otherwise 94–98 %.

Burdens of Oxygen Therapy

Carbon dioxide retention is a key risk, and has been described in patients with COPD, asthma, pneumonia and obesity-hypoventilation syndrome. Although conventionally believed to occur because of the loss of hypoxic ventilatory drive, the fact that there is very little reduction in ventilation at a high PaO_2 in patients retaining carbon dioxide has led to the current understanding that the primary mechanism is a worsening of VQ matching. Lung atelectasis, caused by the lack of relatively insoluble nitrogen, may also contribute to carbon dioxide retention. Interestingly, oxygen is more dense and viscous than air, and there is some evidence that it can reduce FEV_1 slightly and therefore potentially may actually increase the work of breathing.

Oxygen therapy may reduce quality of life for a number of reasons:

- *Drying of upper airways*. Oxygen dries the nasopharyngeal mucosa which can cause discomfort and even nasal bleeding. Humidifiers are noisy and ineffective, and run the risk of bacterial contamination.
- *Psychological dependence*. This frequently occurs and patients may become very frightened during even a short interruption in oxygen supply. Such dependence greatly hinders withdrawal of unhelpful oxygen therapy.
- *Social restriction*. The equipment may restrict movement and activities both within the home and outside, contributing to deconditioning. Oxygen, being highly combustible, will prevent entry into rooms with a lit fire or gas cooking equipment. A sense of stigma can also compound social isolation.

Supplemental oxygen is so extensively used that it is one of the most expensive therapies used in the NHS in the UK. The cost of home oxygen alone is £110 million per year. As it has been estimated that up to 75 % of SBOT users could safely have treatment withdrawn after clinical assessment, the potential cost savings could be immense.

Mrs Todd: Part A

Mrs Todd is a 78 year old lady with moderate COPD. She had been coping with her condition well, getting out twice a week to the local shops, and her chest infections responded to antibiotics from her GP. Unfortunately last winter she had required admission to hospital for intravenous antibiotics. Although she did not qualify for LTOT, she was prescribed home oxygen (SBOT) on discharge from hospital as she had been rather breathless with the chest infection.

She was seen at home by a respiratory nurse specialist, Amanda, one month after discharge. Although she had fully recovered from the infection, her mood was low. She could no longer get out to meet her grandchildren in the park opposite her flat. Even cooking had become difficult as she felt very vulnerable taking the oxygen off when she needed to use the gas stove. She had not left the house since discharge from hospital, and had had one or two episodes of panic when she had called an ambulance, although she had not been admitted. She was becoming totally reliant on her husband who, at 85, was becoming exhausted.

Amanda checked Mrs Todd's oxygen saturation and it was 95 % on air. When she suggested that the oxygen may not be necessary, Mrs Todd was furious. "How can you say that, when I'm getting more and more breathless! I need it! It's my life line." Mr Todd was equally frustrated, "The oxygen is the only I can give her when she's feeling bad"

Case continued in part B on page 45

Fan Therapy

A small hand-held fan is a simple, cheap and portable piece of equipment increasingly used by breathless patients, and widely recommended by respiratory and palliative care clinicians. It provides the cooling, fresh air sensation that patients often crave, in a way that is more feasible than continually having to stand by an open window. It could, however, easily be dismissed as 'a childish gadget' rather than a real treatment. What evidence is there for its effectiveness?

Evidence Base

There has long been evidence for the effectiveness of cold facial stimulation in reducing the sensation of breathlessness in healthy volunteers with induced breathlessness (Schwartzstein et al. 1987; Simon et al. 1991). There have subsequently been three controlled trials in breathless patients evaluating the facial cooling induced by a fan.

Research Evidence

- Baltzan et al. (2000) compared oxygen and a fan with oxygen alone during 6-min walk tests in 17 patients with COPD. A small but non-significant reduction in breathlessness was seen on the first day, but not the subsequent two days (Baltzan et al. 2000).
- Galbraith et al. (2010) compared 5 min use of a fan directed to the face with a fan directed to the leg in a cross-over study in 50 patients with mixed cardiopulmonary disease. There was a significant improvement in breathlessness when the fan was directed to the face (Galbraith et al. 2010).
- Bausewein et al. (2010) undertook a phase 2 parallel group feasibility study comparing use of a hand-held fan with pulling on a plastic wrist band in 70 patients with advanced disease. After 2 month 9/23 in the fan

group and 4/11 in the wrist band group found the intervention helpful (Bausewein et al. 2010).

- A rigorous phase 3 mixed-methods study evaluated the effectiveness of the Cambridge Breathlessness Intervention Service. As well as proving cost-effectiveness for the intervention as a whole, the qualitative data showed that the fan and careful teaching about its use, was a highly valued core component of the complex intervention (Farquhar et al. Submitted for publication).

Although the evidence of effectiveness from quantitative research is, as yet, inconclusive, the qualitative data is compelling. There is also a growing body of anecdotal evidence; in clinical practice it is clear that patients consistently report benefit from the fan. Can this be reconciled with the controlled trial data? The control in the negative Baltzan study was a flow of oxygen which may have had a 'fan-like' effect and prevented a difference between intervention and control. The Bausewein study was a feasibility study aiming to generate data to optimise the design of a larger definitive study. It lacked statistical power and the use of the fan was not reinforced or supported after the initial contact.

Potential Mechanisms

- *Stimulation of facial and nasopharyngeal receptors.* In 1988, Liss and Grant showed that a cool flow of gas reduces the perception of breathlessness in an effect that can be blocked with local anaesthetic. It may be that this mechanism relates to the diving reflex, where stimulation of cold-sensitive receptors in the nasal cavity and areas supplied by the trigeminal nerve triggers a cascade of events that allows an animal to stay under water without breathing for extended periods.
- *Placebo effect.* It is conceivable that patients' belief that the fan is a helpful intervention could be leading to a

placebo effect. Anecdotally, giving patients a fan with a careful explanation for how it appears to work and how exactly to use it, seems to lead to more reliable benefit than simply handing over a fan with minimal explanation.

Clinical Guideline for Use of a Handheld Fan

> "... tiny but so effective ... brilliant ... definitely it does seem to work" (Booth et al. 2006)

The fan is perceived by patients as one of the most important treatment strategies for the management of intractable breathlessness. Although the evidence base is not conclusive, it is clear that patients benefit from it, whatever the mechanism. Given that it is entirely safe and cheap, and that it gives patients control and supports self-management, there is no reason not to offer a fan to every patient requiring palliation of breathlessness.

This guidance does not, therefore, relate to whether or not the fan should be offered. Given that the quality of the explanation when introducing the fan seems to impact on its effectiveness, it is important to consider *how*, rather than when, to use the fan.

- Explain that the fan eases breathlessness, and particularly helps shorten recovery time after exertion. It forms an important part of the 'recovery breathing technique' (chapter 5, page 99)
- Outline scientific evidence supporting use of the fan, adapting the words chosen, to suit the individual patient). Patients usually appreciate knowing that it is a formal treatment that has been researched, and that there is some evidence that it works through cooling the nose and mouth. This feeds back information to the brain that alters the sensation of breathlessness.
- Encourage the patient (rather than a carer) to hold the fan about 15–20 cm or 6–8 in. from the face, directed at the nose and mouth. It usually works within a few minutes.

- Manage a blocked nose or dry mouth, for example with steroid nose drops or artificial saliva. Consistent with its presumed mechanism of action, the fan appears to be less effective in such conditions.
- Encourage patients to take the fan with them when they are out, and to keep a few in different parts of the house so that they do not need to search for one at home.
- Emphasise how the fan can help a person stay in control, rather than simply waiting helplessly for an attack of breathlessness. Encourage patients to use early rather than when they have become very breathless.
- Finally, actually demonstrate use of the fan with the patient during the meeting, reinforcing where to hold it. Patients often get an immediate sense of relief, as they may be experiencing a degree of breathlessness from prolonged talking with the healthcare professional.

Small hand-held fans are widely available and very cheap. Three bladed fans may be more effective than those with two blades as the current of air is stronger.

Are there any disadvantages to using the fan? Some patients do not need a fan, particularly when the breathlessness is mild and the patient has other effective strategies to shorten recovery time. Occasionally patients resist using the fan in public places as it may lead to unwanted attention or cause embarrassment. Sometimes patients are concerned about feeling cold. This is certainly problem with the draughts caused by a room fan but, as long as the rest of the body is warm, a small fan directed at the nose and mouth tends not to cause people to feel uncomfortably cold.

Facial cooling can also be achieved with a damp face cloth, wet-wipe or water mist spray. Anecdotally, this appears to be more acceptable to a small number of patients.

Key Points

- In most patients, oxygen does not palliate breathlessness. Its use should be reserved for severely hypoxaemic patients, and for the few patients who benefit during an individual clinical assessment. Oxygen therapy is burdensome and leads to dependence.
- A small hand-held fan tends to be more effective. It is cheap and entirely safe, gives patients control, and promotes self-management and independence.
- The fan is one of the most important strategies in the palliation of breathlessness in advanced disease.

Mrs Todd: Part B **(continued from page 40)**

Mrs Todd and her husband were clearly not going to accept withdrawal of oxygen therapy. Amanda, her respiratory nurse, felt deeply frustrated as she knew the oxygen was unlikely to be indicated, given her good oxygen saturation, and it was causing so many problems. The restriction of activity meant she was becoming deconditioned and more breathless; she was getting increasingly anxious about managing without the oxygen and had even had some panic attacks. Even her husband, with his increasing sense of helplessness, was becoming reliant on her using it.

Amanda realised that the only way forward would be to gain Mr and Mrs Todd's trust through other approaches. Mrs Todd did realise she was uncharacteristically tense and anxious at the moment, and listened carefully to the explanation of how this could influence her breathing. She was keen to learn to relax and accepted a CD with a guided imagery narrative. Amanda also introduced the hand-held fan, carefully explaining how it is believed to work. Having emphasised her good oxygen saturation reading, she planted the idea in Mrs Todd's mind that much of the benefit of oxygen therapy may occur because of the 'fan effect', a cool flow of gas.

By the next meeting, Mrs Todd's situation had begun to improve. She had found the fan helpful, and was open to the suggestion that she could try to reduce the time she used the oxygen, and would use the fan in its place. They agreed a programme of weaning the oxygen, with regular telephone contact from Amanda. Within 2 weeks, she had successfully almost entirely stopped using the oxygen. She could now get out of the house, with the fan always in her pocket, and she was gradually building up the distance she could walk outside. Mr Todd, too, felt relieved that by passing her the fan, he had something he could 'do', when his wife was acutely breathless. It made him feel less frightened himself and more in control.

The last time they met, Mrs Todd was delighted; she had made it right across the park with her grandchildren beside her. When Amanda suggested giving back the oxygen equipment, Mrs Todd laughed, "That might just be step to far … but, you know, that fan is just great …"

References

Abernethy A, McDonald C, Frith P, et al. Effect of palliative oxygen versus room air in relief of breathlessness in patients with refractory dyspnoea: a double-blind, randomised controlled trial. Lancet. 2010;376:784–93.

Baltzan M, Alter A, Rotaple M, Kamel H, Wolkove N. Fan to palliative exercise-induced dyspnoea with severe COPD. Am J Respir Crit Care Med. 2000;161(3 Suppl):A59.

Bausewein C, Booth S, Gysels M, Kuhnbach R, Higginson I. Effectiveness of a hand-held fan for breathlessness: a randomised phase II trial. BMC Palliat Care. 2010;9:22.

Booth S, Kelly MJ, Cox NP, et al. Does oxygen help dyspnea in patients with cancer? Am J Respir Crit Care Med. 1996;153:1515–8.

Booth S, Farquhar M, Gysels M, Bausewein C, Higginson IJ. The impact of a breathlessness intervention service (BIS) on the lives of patients with intractable dyspnoea: a qualitative. Phase I study. Palliat Support Care. 2006;4:287–93.

Farquhar M, Prevost A, McCrone P et al. Is a specialist breathlessness service more effective for patients with advanced cancer and their carers than standard care? Findings of a mixed method randomised controlled trial. Submitted for publication.

Galbraith S, Fagan P, Perkins P, Lynch A, Booth S. Does the use of a handheld fan improve chronic dyspnea? A randomised, controlled, cross-over trial. J Pain Symptom Manage. 2010;39(5):831–8.

Liss H, Grant B. The effect of nasal flow on breathlessness in patients with chronic obstructive pulmonary disease. Am Rev Respir Dis. 1988;137:1285–8.

Moore R, Berlowitz D, Denehy L, et al. A randomised trial of domiciliary, ambulatory oxygen in patients with COPD and dyspnoea but without resting hypoxaemia. Thorax. 2011;66:32–7.

Schwartzstein R, Lahive K, Pope A, et al. Cold facial stimulation reduces breathlessness induced in normal subjects. Am Rev Respir Dis. 1987;136:58–61.

Simon P, Basner R, Weinberger S, et al. Oral mucosal stimulation modulates intensity of breathlessness induced in normal subjects. Am Rev Respir Dis. 1991;144(2):419–22.

Spathis A, Booth S. End of life care in chronic obstructive pulmonary disease. Int J Chron Obstruct Pulmon Dis. 2008;3(1):11–29.

Uronis H, Currow D, McCrory D, Samsa G, Abernethy A. Oxygen for relief of dyspnoea in mildly- or non-hypoxaemic patients with cancer: a systematic review and meta-analysis. Br J Cancer. 2008;98:294–9.

Uronis H, McCrory D, Samsa G, Currow D, Abernethy A. Symptom oxygen for non-hypoxaemic chronic obstructive pulmonary disease. Cochrane Database Syst Rev. 2011;(6); Art. No.: CD006429.

Chapter 4
Positions to Ease Breathlessness

Getting my breath back with this kind of position, leaning on my elbows, that was a very useful suggestion

– A gentleman with pulmonary fibrosis.

Introduction

Positions to ease breathlessness are often used in conjunction with breathing techniques and facial cooling using a fan, wet flannel or cold spray. The forward lean position and passively fixing the shoulder girdle is recommended in the British Thoracic Society and Association of Chartered Physiotherapists in Respiratory Care (BTS/ACPRC) (2009) guidelines to help ease breathlessness in those with COPD, although the evidence base is not strong as positioning has not been a topic of research interest in recent times.

Positions of ease are often taken up instinctively by patients when breathless. It may reassure patients to know that similar positions are used by athletes to ease breathlessness after finishing a race. Patients usually select the most appropriate position for them, therefore, as part of their assessment, clinicians should ask patients if they have found certain positions help ease their breathing.

Providing Advice on Positioning

- Suggest a patient tries a position of ease, if they are do not already use one

S. Booth et al., *Managing Breathlessness in Clinical Practice*,
DOI 10.1007/978-1-4471-4754-1_4,

- Explain how and why certain positions may ease breathlessness, therefore improving the patient and carers confidence in managing breathlessness.
- If a patient instinctively uses a position of ease offer modifications that may improve the position's effectiveness.
- Suggest alternative positions for different situations.
- Where appropriate, suggest and explain the use of walking aids to improve the effectiveness of breathing muscles and therefore ease breathlessness when mobilising.
- Suggest positions for breathlessness at rest.

Forward Lean

The diaphragm is the primary muscle of inspiration. It is believed that a forward lean position helps to dome the diaphragm, lengthening its muscle fibres, improving the length-tension relationship and therefore improving its force generating and ventilatory capacity (O'Neill and McCarthy 1983; Sharp et al. 1980; Barach 1974). The accessory muscles of exhalation, which include the abdominals (Fig. 4.1), may also be placed in an improved position for contraction by some degree of forward lean.

Doming the diaphragm with forward lean is thought to be of particular benefit to those with obstructive lung disease such as COPD or emphysema who have hyperinflated lungs and therefore their diaphragm is in a shortened position. However patients with very severe hyperinflation with extremely flattened diaphragms may prefer a less flexed position to avoid 'fixing' the diaphragm between the abdominal contents and hyperinflated lung. Such patients may prefer to focus on positions that fix the upper limbs to improve inspiratory accessory muscle efficiency.

In milder episodes of breathlessness forward lean alone, as in Fig. 4.2, may be enough to ease breathing through doming of the diaphragm and perhaps improved abdominal muscle contraction.

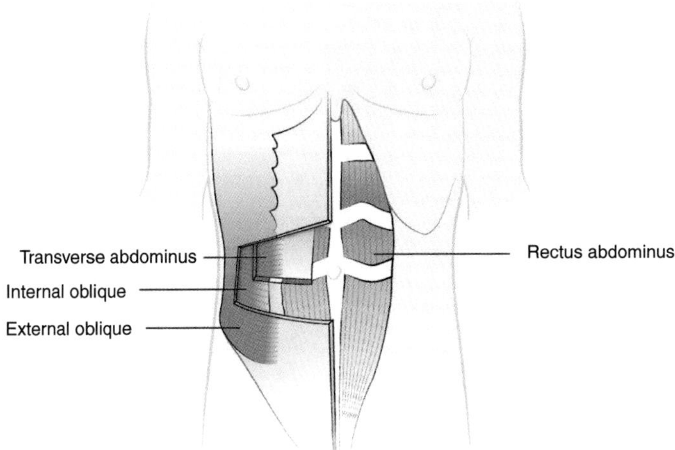

FIGURE 4.1 Abdominal muscles, the accessory muscles of expiration © CBIS, 2013

Leaning vs Bending from the Waist

> *It's weird ... I can go for a walk ... several hundred yards ... breathless up to a point and yet ... I like bend ... and then I start the breathlessness. It's very unpleasant ... suffocation.*
>
> – Gentleman with lung cancer.

It is worth noting that the forward lean position is just a lean from the waist and not a full bend. Patients often find bending fully, for example when picking up an item from the floor or putting on their socks and shoes, actually increases their feeling of breathlessness, no matter what the pathology. This is especially true for patients who have very hyperinflated lungs or those with large or tight abdomens. Bending fully may cause the abdominal contents to push up against and obstruct the downward movement of the diaphragm during inspiration. A rational explanation as to why breathlessness is increased when bending down may help to reduce patient anxiety. This explanation may also open up conversation regarding the use of long handled aids to assist with activities of daily living and avoid bending.

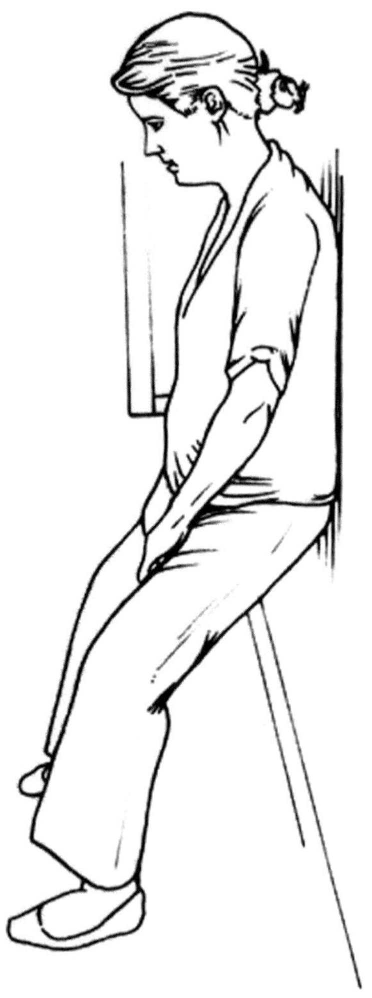

FIGURE 4.2 Forward lean with back against wall © CBIS, 2013

Fixation of the Shoulder Girdle

Banzett et al. (1988) showed that improved ventilatory capacity occurred when 'normals' brace their arms.

> It is thought that fixing the shoulder girdle improves the length-tension relationship of muscles that attach between the ribs and the upper limb or shoulder girdle therefore improving their capacity to act as breathing accessory muscles.

In addition, instead of having the rib cage as the fixed point and moving the limb as in normal arm use; the limb is fixed and therefore the effect of the muscle's pull can be transferred to the ribs to aid respiration. The BTS/ACPRC (2009) guidelines suggest that shoulder girdle fixation should be passive as this may help reduce oxygen consumption. Inspiratory breathing accessory muscles that may aid respiration through shoulder girdle fixation are shown in Figs. 4.3 and 4.4.

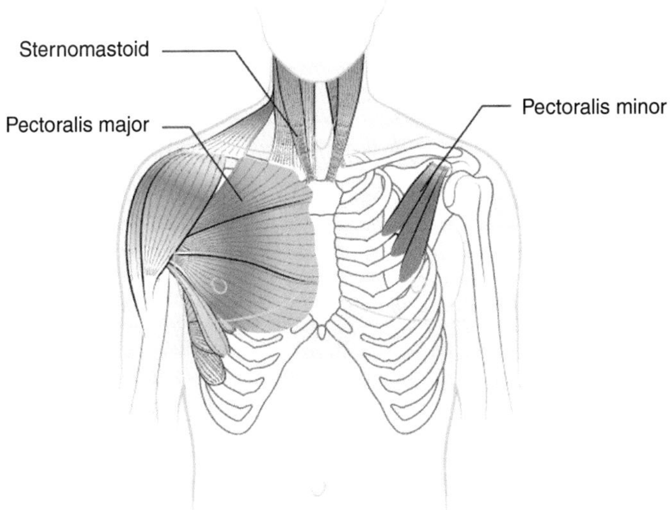

FIGURE 4.3 Anterior breathing accessory muscles © CBIS, 2013

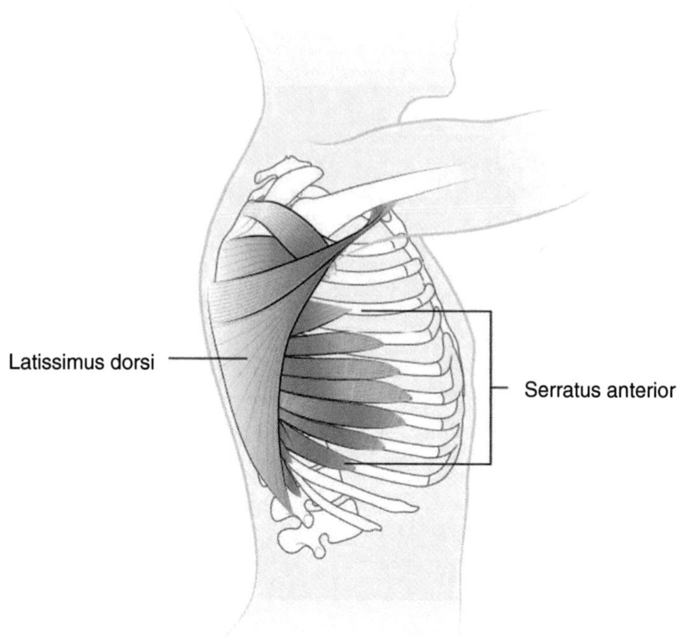

FIGURE 4.4 Posterior inspiratory breathing accessory muscles © CBIS, 2013

Sternomastoid is also widely recognised an inspiratory accessory muscle, helping to pull on the sternum and increase the 'pump handle' movement of the chest during effortful breathing. The scalenes were traditionally thought to be accessory muscles and only active during effortful breathing, however evidence is now emerging that the scalenes rhythmically contract in time with respiration during relaxed breathing in 'normals' and are therefore primary muscles of inspiration.

The muscles of the posterior chest wall (Fig. 4.4) such as serratus anterior and latissimus dorsi aid respiration in a similar way, augmented through bracing of the shoulder girdle and upper limb. It has been debated as to whether all the

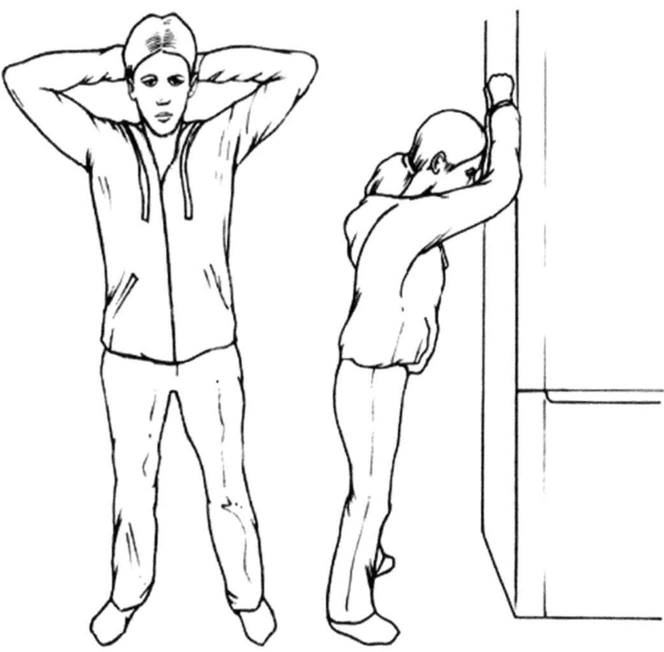

FIGURE 4.5 Upper limb bracing with elevation © CBIS, 2013

fibres of these large muscles are aligned correctly to aid respiration however their length-tension relationship as well as the direction of pull may be more effective on the ribs when the upper limb is fixed in an elevated position. Positions that particularly augment rib pull by both anterior and posterior chest wall muscles are shown in Fig. 4.5.

In milder episodes of breathlessness bracing of the upper limbs alone may be sufficient to ease breathing (Fig. 4.6).

> Less conspicuous ways to brace the upper limbs and shoulder girdle include placing the hands or thumbs in or on pockets, belt loops, waistband or handbag strap.

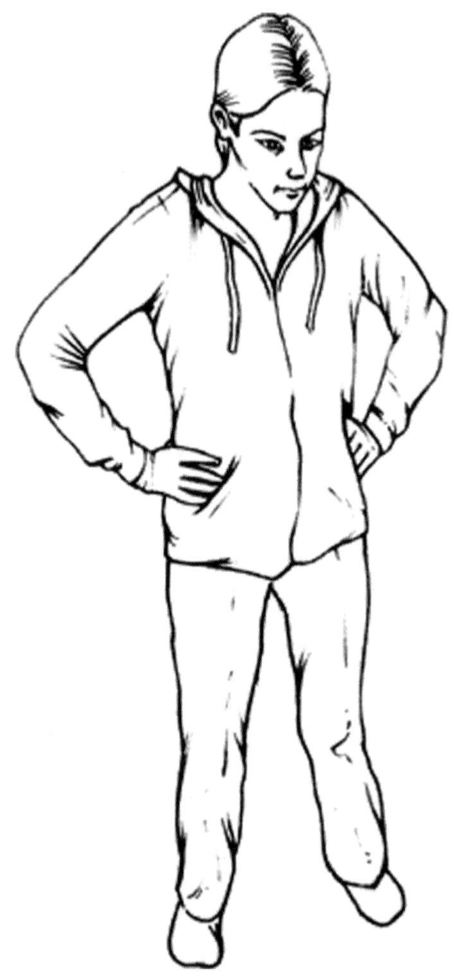

FIGURE 4.6 'Hands on hips', upper limb bracing © CBIS, 2013

Combining Forward Lean with Upper Limb Bracing

Positions of ease that maybe explained by both the forward lean's effect on the diaphragm and upper limb bracing theory are shown in Fig. 4.7.

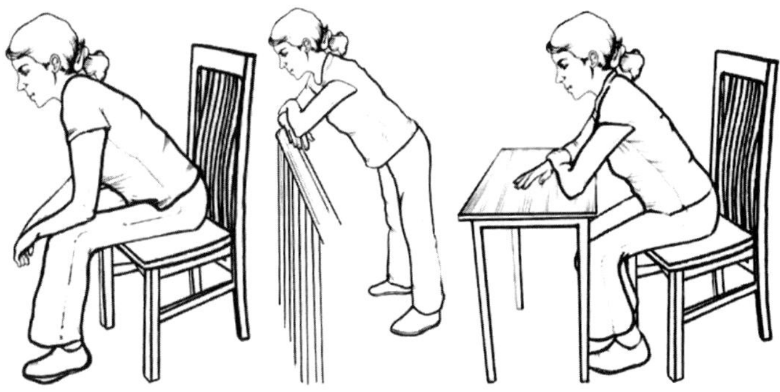

FIGURE 4.7 Combined forward lean with upper limb bracing © CBIS, 2013

Patients often report the effectiveness of these positions is improved by allowing hands to be open and relaxed, their wrists, shoulders and neck to relax and their legs to be apart.

Patients with a large or tight abdomen may actually find they recover quicker with a forward lean position in standing compared to sitting as the standing position produces less compression on their abdomen, thus imposing less restriction on their diaphragm. If a patient with a large or tight abdomen prefers to sit to recover their breathing then sitting on a higher seat such as a perching stool, having their elbows straight when bracing their hands on their knees and having their legs apart may reduce the splinting of the diaphragm by the abdominal contents.

Explaining How Positioning Works to Patients and Carers

(Include physical demonstration as you explain)

When an athlete finishes a race you may have noticed them bending forward with their hand on their knees as they try to recover their breathing. In a similar way you may have noticed leaning forward and bracing on your arms helps you to recover from breathlessness. The athlete's breathlessness and your breathlessness are the same but it takes a lot more exercise to make the athlete breathless. It is instinctive to take up this forward lean position when breathless as the body knows what to do for the best. By fixing your arms still, muscles around the upper chest and shoulder, that usually move your arm, can pull at their other end and pull on the ribs instead and therefore help with breathing.

Leaning forward also helps to dome the large, flat diaphragm muscle so it has the ability to move down further and draw in more air.

Upper Limb Activity

It is common for breathlessness to be aggravated by lifting and carrying objects, such as shopping bags, or doing activities with the upper limb above the head, such as washing the hair. There are a number of factors which cause breathlessness to increase in such situations, such as increased work load of the heart and lungs. However such upper limb activity may also inhibit the ability of the breathing accessory muscles aid inspiration as these muscles are being asked to both stabilise the shoulder girdle, move the arm and pull on the ribs all at the same time. Education as to why such activities may make a patient feel more breathless may help reduce anxiety by providing a rational explanation. This can then lead into a conversation regarding the use of long handled aids to help daily living or the use of personal shopping trolleys to avoid carrying bags.

Walking Aids

The use of walking aids to ease exertional breathlessness is recommended in BTS/ACPRC (2009) guidelines, with a stronger evidence base than static positioning. Significant improvement in walking distance and ventilatory capacity has been seen in those with COPD when using a rollator

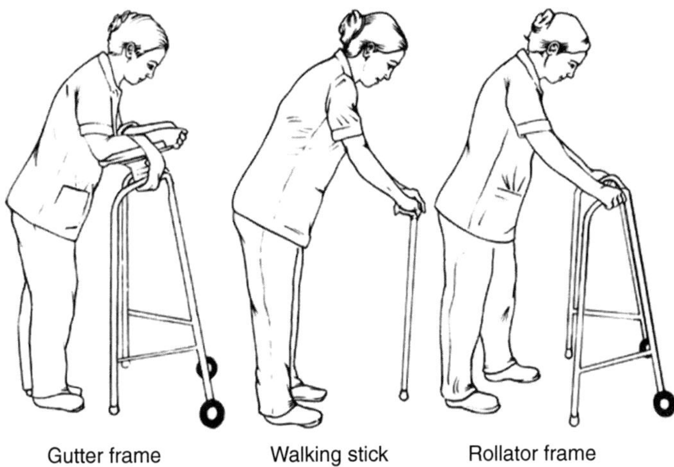

FIGURE 4.8 Use of walking aids to ease exertional breathlessness © CBIS, 2013

frame (Probst et al. 2004). This may explain way patients often report being able to walk further within a supermarket pushing a supermarket trolley. Browsing supermarket shelves also provides patients with the socially acceptable excuse to walk slowly and to stop to rest at regular intervals, therefore making them feel less self conscious when trying to pace themselves. It may therefore be appropriate to encourage patients to regularly walk the isles of the supermarket pushing a trolley as part of an exercise routine.

The use of a walking aid allows patients to 'take the forward lean position with them' as they walk therefore improving the efficiency of their breathing muscles during this activity. Using a walking aid has the additional benefit of slowing down a patient who tends to rush. It also provides a portable leaning post, which may boost the confidence of a more anxious patient, especially in the wide open spaces of the hospital or hospice environment or when walking outside the house. Of course the use of walking aids maybe just as appropriate within the home.

There are a variety of walking aids available (Fig. 4.8). The 'gutter framc' provides the most support and allows passive shoulder girdle fixation when stopping to rest, however gutter frames can be awkward to manoeuvre and are therefore not always practical. A walking stick provides an intermittent leaning post rather than continual support. A walking stick maybe more acceptable to a patient who is reluctant to try a walking aid to help them manage their breathlessness. Some walking sticks are designed so that they can transform into a portable seat, which may benefit some patients. The wheels of a rollator frame reduce energy expenditure as the patient does not have to lift the frame with each step. Gutter and rollator frames are not designed for outdoor use as they can be unstable on uneven ground. Three or four wheeled walkers are more suitable for use outdoors. Four wheeled walkers are more stable than three wheeled walkers and may also come with a seat with storage space beneath providing additional benefits to the patient. Three wheeled walkers maybe easier than four wheeled walkers to fold and store.

Positions for Breathlessness at Rest

A patient may experience significant breathlessness at rest near end of life or during an exacerbation of their condition. When a patient is breathless at rest they may be unable to obtain a comfortable position independently therefore relatives, carers, hospital or hospice staff may have to assist the patient to achieve an optimal position for their breathing. The role of the clinician will therefore not only be to educate the patient but also the carers and staff. Patients who are breathless at rest are at risk of fatigue. The following positions therefore have the duel aim of improving the efficiency of the breathing muscles while supporting the patient's position as much as possible, reducing energy expenditure and therefore reducing fatigue.

Supported Forward Lean in Sitting

Supported forward lean in sitting may improve the efficiency of the diaphragm and accessory muscles, while supporting the patient in such a way that they have to expend little energy to

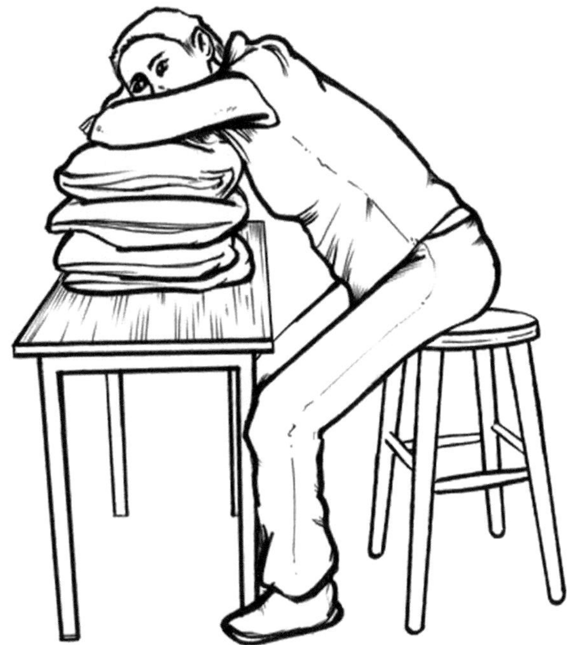

FIGURE 4.9 Supported forward lean in sitting © CBIS, 2013

maintain the position (Fig. 4.9). This position is often favoured by asthmatics during an acute attack but may also be beneficial for others who are breathless at rest. Having the legs apart and sitting on a higher seat or raised bed may also help to remove abdominal restriction from the diaphragm. This is especially important if the abdomen is large or tight. Patients who are breathless when sitting on the toilet may find leaning onto a walking frame or a back of a chair with a pillow on top for comfort enables them to achieve this position.

Supported Sitting

Supported sitting can be achieved in a comfortable chair or in long sitting on a bed, with legs out in front. Pillows are placed under the head and forearms to support the weight of the head and arms, therefore reducing energy expenditure and helping the shoulders and neck to relax. Remember pillows can be very insulating and surrounding a patient with pillows may cause them to become uncomfortably hot, increasing their respiratory rate and therefore their breathlessness. Comfort maybe improved by a pillow under the knees in long sitting. If the patient's feet do not reach the floor when sitting in a chair then a block under their feet maybe required.

Adjusting a profiling bed to a 'chair' position maybe a comfortable position when breathless as it allows an upright position without overly flexing the patient at the abdomen, which would restrict the diaphragm. The 'chair' position may be achieved by elevating the foot end of the bed as far as possible, this is to prevent the patient sliding down the bed. The head of the bed is then elevated, but not fully, perhaps to about 45°. The whole bed can then be tilted feet down to gain further elevation of the head without flexing at the abdomen.

High Side Lying

High side lying can be a very comfortable position for the breathless patient (Fig. 4.10). It is important the patient is positioned fully onto their side as this will allow the abdominal contents to move away from the diaphragm and therefore not restrict its movement. For this reason side lying can be particularly comfortable for patients with large or tight abdomens. The patient can be encouraged to relax the upper most upper limb onto the pillows and therefore relax the shoulder girdle as much as able. If comfortable, some patients find having their upper most arm flexed at the shoulder, so the arm rests close to the head, encourages an opening of the rib cage on this side and perhaps improve the line of pull of breathing accessory muscles, therefore easing breathlessness further. The head is fully supported allowing the neck to relax. As with the supported long sitting position, with a profiling bed

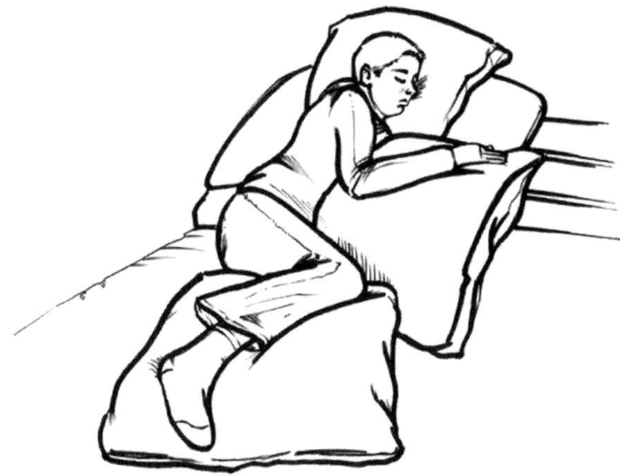

FIGURE 4.10 High side lying © CBIS, 2013

the feet can be elevated as much as comfortable, to avoid the patient slipping down the bed. The head can then be elevated slightly before tilting the whole bed feet down to elevate the head further without flexing the patient at the waist and compressing their abdomen.

Summary

Positions to ease breathlessness empower the patient to manage their own symptoms. Even though patients often take up effective and appropriate positions instinctively the clinician's knowledge and skill in explaining why such positions ease breathlessness improves the patient's confidence in their ability to self manage. Clinicians should suggest appropriate positions to patients who do not instinctively use them and modifications, if required, to improve effectiveness of a position instinctively used. Clinicians should also consider suggesting the use of walking aids to help manage exertional breathlessness during mobilisation.

Remember to always ask the patient what position works for them. Don't assume the 'textbook answer' is always right!

Unique positions of ease adopted by patients

"To help relax my breathing as I fall asleep I place a pillow on my chest and rest my arms on top of it- Lady with COPD."

"My breathing feels easier when I lie on the sofa on my right side, with my left arm above my head. I often watch TV like this - Gentleman with severe emphysema"

"If I feel breathless at night I reach behind my head and hold the head board of my bed until my breathing eases- Lady with moderate COPD"

"To get my breath back after mowing the lawn I hold onto a high window ledge above my head- Gentleman with moderate COPD"

"To ease my breathing I sit on my arm chair and reach behind my head to hold the back of the chair- Gentleman with Lung cancer and COPD"

Key Points

- Positioning improves the efficiency and effectiveness of both primary and accessory muscles of breathing
- Breathless patients often instinctively take up appropriate and effective positions of ease
- Clinicians should suggest appropriate positions of ease to breathless patients who do not use instinctive positioning
- Where appropriate, clinicians should suggest modifications to improve the effectiveness of instinctive positions
- It is important to explain why positions of ease help to reduce breathlessness as this improves the patient's confidence in their use.
- Walking aids should be considered to enable positions of ease to be used during mobilising to help reduce exertional breathlessness

References

Banzett RB, Topulos GP, Leith DE, et al. Bracing arms increases the capacity for sustained hyperpnoea. Am Rev Respir Dis. 1988;138: 106–9.

Barach AL. Chronic obstructive lung disease: postural relief of dyspnoea. Arch Phys Med Rehabil. 1974;55:494–504.

British Thoracic Society (BTS) & Association of Chartered Physiotherapists in Respiratory Care (ACPRC). Guidelines for the physiotherapy management of the adult, medical, spontaneously breathing patient. Thorax. 2009;64(Supplement I):i1–51.

O'Neill S, McCarthy DS. Postural relief of dyspnoea in severe chronic airflow limitation: relationship to respiratory muscle strength. Thorax. 1983;38:595–600.

Probst VS, Trooster T, Coosemans I, Spruit MA, de Oliveira Pitta F, Decramer M, Gosselink R. Mechanisms of improvement in exercise capacity using a rollator in patients with COPD. Chest. 2004;126: 1102–7.

Sharp JT, Drutz WS, Moisan T, et al. Postural relief of dyspnoea in severe chronic obstructive pulmonary disease. Am Rev Respir Dis. 1980;122: 201–11.

Chapter 5
Breathing Techniques for Breathlessness

My doctor said you would teach me how to breathe correctly.
What a ridiculous idea, I have been breathing all my life!
– A patient's view on breathing techniques.

Introduction

Breathing techniques are most commonly used in combination with positioning and the fan to the face or other facial cooling. This chapter will focus on three different breathing techniques that can help reduce the feeling of breathlessness:

- Breathing Control
- Pursed-lips Breathing
- Recovery Breathing

Technique selection, modification to suit the patient and combining techniques will be discussed, as well as the role of breathing pattern re-education in breathlessness management.

Breathing Control vs Diaphragmatic Breathing

The terms Breathing Control and Diaphragmatic Breathing are often used interchangeably however the British Thoracic Society and Association of Chartered Physiotherapists in

S. Booth et al., *Managing Breathlessness in Clinical Practice*,
DOI 10.1007/978-1-4471-4754-1_5,

Respiratory Care (BTS/ACPRC) (2009) guidelines (p. i49) offer the following two different definitions:

Breathing Control
"Normal tidal breathing encouraging relaxation of the upper chest and shoulders."

Diaphragmatic Breathing
"Breathing using abdominal movement, reducing the degree of chest wall movement as much as possible."

The key difference between Breathing Control and Diaphragmatic Breathing is the volume of air taken in on each breath. Breathing Control advocates "**normal tidal breathing**" i.e. bringing breathing back to normal tidal volume. Diaphragmatic breathing has been described to be a long, slow, deep inspiration, similar to breathing techniques used in Yoga, Tai Chi and other complementary therapies with the aim to deliberately increase tidal volume and slow respiratory rate. However the differentiation of Diaphragmatic Breathing from Breathing Control is not universally recognised and these terms are sometimes used interchangeably.

In severe Chronic Obstructive Pulmonary Disease (COPD) deliberately increasing tidal volume may increase lung hyperinflation causing asynchronous rib cage movement, uneven distribution of air within the lungs and therefore increase the work of breathing and dyspnoea (Vitacca et al. 1998; Gosselink et al. 1995).

This led the BTS/ACPRC (2009) guidelines to recommend that Diaphragmatic Breathing is not advocated for patients with hyperinflation and should not be taught routinely to patients with severe COPD.

Breathing Control: Efficient Breathing

> *"Sitting, with my hand on my tummy and breathing from there. It helps a lot when I am breathless and its very relaxing"*- A patient with COPD.
>
> *"She said don't push your breath out, just let it go, let it relax. I notice I recover very quickly now by doing this when breathless"* – A patient with lung cancer.

A trial of Breathing Control has been recommended for the management of breathlessness in COPD (BTS/ACPRC 2009). National Institute for Clinical Excellence (NICE) Lung Cancer Guidelines (NICE 2011) suggests Breathing Control should be considered as part of a system of non-pharmacological measures to manage breathlessness.

Breathing Control encourages patients to bring their breathing back to an efficient breathing pattern with the aim to relax the breathing accessory muscles and bring the focus breathing back to the efficient and relatively fatigue resistant diaphragm.

Apart from promoting efficient use of respiratory muscles Breathing Control may also help in the management of breathlessness by reducing the speed of airflow; promoting laminar flow, efficiency of air movement and even distribution of air within the lungs. Breathing Control may deter unnecessary hyperventilation and its associated symptoms by promoting the return of breathing to an appropriate tidal volume and respiratory rate. Dynamic hyperinflation may also be deterred as exhalation is relaxed and lengthened and respiratory rate and tidal volume are controlled. Some patients report Breathing Control to be a relaxing and calming focus when breathless.

TABLE 5.1 Efficient breathing

Appropriate minute volume	Appropriate respiratory rate
	Appropriate tidal volume
Efficient muscle use	Reduce breathing accessory muscle use
	Focus breathing on using the efficient diaphragm
	Expiration is passive at rest and is created by the passive recoil of the lung and thoracic cage. Aim for expiration to be as passive as pathology allows.
Efficient breathing pattern	Expiration is longer than inspiration, with a normal ratio of 1:1.5–2. 'Normal' expiration will be even longer in those with obstructive airways disease.
	End expiratory pause
Nose vs mouth	Nose breathing at rest

When assessing how efficiently a patient is breathing it can help to compare their breathing pattern to the 'ideal' efficient breathing described in Table 5.1.

Patients with a chronic pathology may breathe in a certain way either due to pathological changes, 'bad habits' or reversible causes. Teaching a patient Breathing Control will help them 'undo' bad habits and achieve as efficient breathing as possible in the presence of pathological changes. Reversible causes such as poor posture and tight musculature should also be addressed.

Introducing Breathing Control

For patients to have confidence in a breathing technique they need to understand how it works. Some patients may be very sceptical, while others may feel 'learning how to breathe right' is just what they need. It is therefore important to begin with patient education involving a simple anatomy lesson and explanation regarding how Breathing Control works before teaching the technique its self. Diagrams showing the movement of the diaphragm during breathing and the location of the breathing accessory muscles are a valuable educational tool.

The Diaphragm

The diaphragm does about 95 % of the work of normal, tidal breathing with minimal contribution of the accessory muscles. The diaphragm has a high ratio of fatigue resistant muscles fibres and is the most fatigue resistant of all skeletal muscles. Essentially the diaphragm is designed to contract with every breath throughout our life, just like our heart beating, and does not tire easily.

When learning Breathing Control at rest patients often want to please and strive for large movements of the tummy, creating large inspiratory volumes, when in fact the aim of Breathing Control is to try to return to 'normal' tidal volume breathing. It is therefore worth explaining to patients that the diaphragm only moves down about 1 cm when breathing at rest, the movement at the tummy is therefore very subtle. During exercise the diaphragm may move down up to 10 cm, in normal, healthy lungs (West 2008).

Breathing Accessory Muscles

Breathing accessory muscles are muscles that assist with breathing when the work of breathing increases (Fig. 5.1). Any muscle that attaches to the ribs or sternum has the potential to be a breathing accessory muscle, if the angle of pull is correct. It is normal to use the breathing accessory muscles when breathless, whether you are a marathon runner or a person with a chronic pathology who becomes breathless just walking across the room. The primary role of the inspiratory accessory muscles (Fig. 5.1a, b) is to move the upper limbs and stabilise the shoulder girdle, not to contract on every breath. For this reason they can become fatigued if used to aid breathing for longer than necessary. It is therefore important to try to bring the breathing focus back to the efficient diaphragm as quickly as possible to help recovery from breathlessness.

The abdominal muscles are the expiratory accessory muscles (Fig. 5.1c) that contract to help push the diaphragm up and expel the air from the lungs when the work of breathing

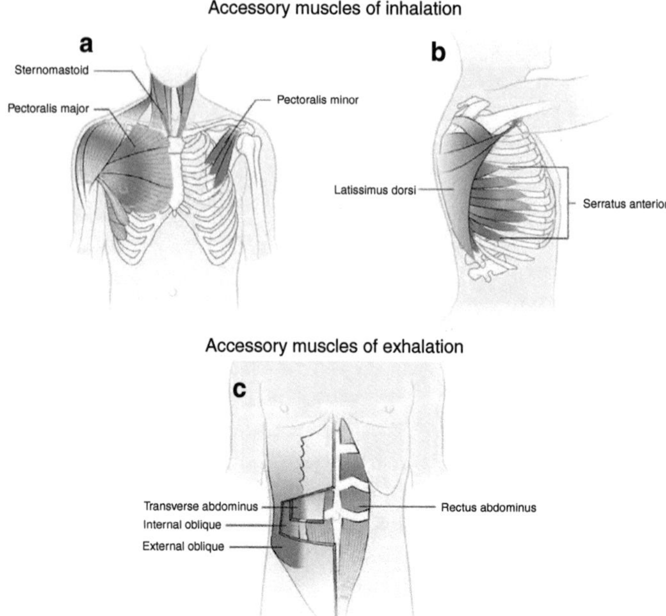

FIGURE 5.1 Breathing accessory muscles © CBIS, 2013. (**a**) Anterior accessory muscles of inhalation. (**b**) Posterior accessory muscles of inhalation. (**c**) Accessory muscles of exhalation

is increased due to pathology or exertion. Expiratory accessory muscles maybe used particularly by those with those with obstructive lung disease who struggle to release air from their lungs. These muscles also fatigue easily and should be encouraged to relax when no longer required to aid breathing.

The Breathing Action of the Diaphragm

Everyone has a preferred learning style. Aids to learning include:

- Verbal description
- Diagrams

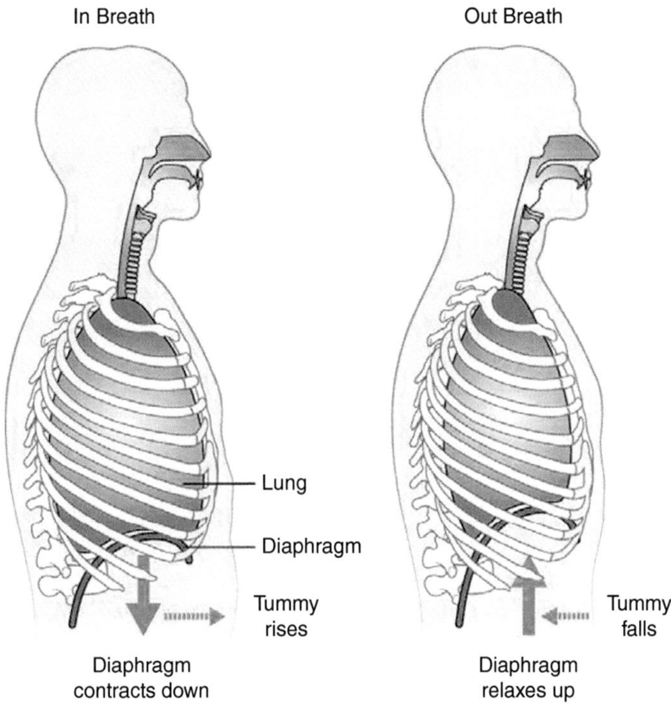

FIGURE 5.2 Diaphragm movement during normal breathing © CBIS, 2013

- Demonstration
- Experiencing for themselves

When teaching a breathing technique it is important to include a variety of teaching styles to try to suit the patient's needs. Try not to overload the patient with too much detail, although some patients maybe fascinated and want more information.

The movement of the diaphragm cannot be felt directly. In order for the patient to link the movement they feel at the tummy with the action of the diaphragm it is important they understand the movement of the diaphragm during normal breathing. The movement of the diaphragm maybe shown through diagrams (Fig. 5.2), demonstration and patient experience.

Demonstrating the Movement of the Diaphragm

1. Clinician holds a domed A4 piece of paper at their own tummy, flattening it as they breathe in and doming it as they breathe out.
2. Clinician puts their hand on their own tummy and exaggerates the breathing movement at the tummy, with the tummy expanding as they breathe in and falling as they breathe out.
3. Patient places their own hand between umbilicus and lower ribs and feels the movement for themselves, under the clinician's guidance.

If the patient is struggling to feel this movement they may find it useful for you to put your hand on their tummy (with or without their hand) and describe the movement as you feel it.

It may also help to describe the abdomen as a box with the diaphragm as the ceiling, the tummy muscles as the walls and the pelvic floor as the floor. As the ceiling (diaphragm) comes down as you breathe in, the walls (tummy muscles) bulge outwards. It is therefore important to keep the walls (tummy muscles) soft and relaxed when learning Breathing Control otherwise it will be difficult to feel the breathing movement. This is why positioning and general relaxation are important first steps in learning Breathing Control. This is to promote relaxation of the abdominal muscles, which are also the expiratory accessory muscles and therefore may be hyperactive from overuse and also to help relax the inspiratory accessory muscles around the neck, shoulders and upper chest so the breathing focus can come more naturally from the tummy, without the upper chest dominating.

Explaining Breathing Control to Patients and Carers

"When someone is very breathless they tend to breathe from the top of their chest. This is a normal thing to do when breathless whether you are an athlete at the end of a race or someone who has a medical condition that makes them feel breathless. When you breathe from the top of your chest you are using the breathing accessory muscles. These are muscles around your upper chest and shoulders that usually move your arms. When you are very breathless these muscles can pull on your ribs and help with breathing.

Unfortunately these upper chest muscles are not designed to help with breathing long term. They get tired easily and may become tight and sore from overuse. It is therefore important to breathing your breathing back to your tummy as soon as you are able. This focuses the breathing back to the strong, efficient diaphragm that is designed for breathing and does not tire easily. It takes less effort to breathe from your diaphragm and so your breathlessness should ease.

Try to breathe from you tummy, with your shoulders relaxed, when you are up and active. This may help you reduce the breathlessness you feel when on the move".

When to Use Breathing Control

Breathing Control is most commonly used to help recover from breathlessness, no matter what the pathological cause. It is important to also consider its use during activity and exercise to try to keep breathing as efficient as possible and avoid hyperventilation. Breathing 'from the tummy' does not often come easily and therefore Breathing Control requires regular practice at rest in order to become familiar with the technique so it can be used effectively when breathless. Regular practice of Breathing Control at rest promotes general relaxation and may also help avoid development, or aid correction, of habitual inefficient breathing patterns.

Teaching Breathing Control

"Now they have taught me to breathe from my stomach.... instead of up here........ They are a great help, especially learning to breathe from here and breathing in and out" – Gentleman with Pulmonary Fibrosis

> The term Breathing Control implies effort and forceful control over breathing when in fact the opposite is true.

When learning Breathing Control the more effort a patient puts into 'getting it right' often the worse the breathing pattern becomes. The term 'relaxed tummy breathing' better reflects the aim of the technique and is more easily understood by patients. The focus should therefore be on relaxation of the body, particularly the neck, shoulders and upper chest ensuring the breathing accessory muscles relax and 'let go'. The patient should 'notice' the movement of the abdomen, rather than make it happen.

Breathing Control may sound simple but can be quite complicated to achieve especially in a breathless, anxious patient who may have experienced breathlessness over a number of years. 'Bad habits' and misconceptions about breathing can form. It is the clinician's skill to see what maybe improved about a patient's breathing pattern i.e. what is habit, poor posture, tight, over active muscles, anxiety or misunderstanding and thus can be changed with practice; and what is pathology driven and cannot be changed. Often a stepwise process to achieving efficient breathing can help to unravel why a patient breathes the way that they do (Table 5.2).

These steps are to help guide the teaching of Breathing Control and retrain breathing patterns. Some patients may mange to move through all these steps in one session, however most patients will require a number of sessions to work through each step. Go at the patient's own pace and try not to

TABLE 5.2 The steps of teaching Breathing Control

Step	Description	Aim
1	Position & Posture	Adjust position and posture to encourage correct breathing muscle use and to promote comfort and relaxation.
	Relax body and mind	Relax the body, especially breathing accessory muscles of inspiration (neck, shoulders and upper chest) and exhalation (abdominal muscles). Reduce accessory muscle use as much as able. Nose breathe, if able and comfortable.
2	Feel the breath	'Tune into' how breathing feels without trying to change anything.
	Notice the tummy rise as you breathe in	Noticing and recognise the action of the diaphragm on the tummy as you breathe.
	Notice the tummy fall as you breathe out	
3	Float the air in, relax the breath out	Achieve normal tidal volume. Take in just the air you need. Make exhalation as passive as possible. Expiration may lengthen and respiratory rate may slow. Expiration should be longer than inspiration.
	Quiet, gentle breaths	Slow inspiratory flow, promote smooth, laminar flow within the airways to reduce turbulence and resistance. Respiratory rate may slow and tidal volume may reduce.
4	Notice the natural pause after the breath out	Notice the pause but do not try to change it. Be comfortable with it.
	Rest in this pause, wait for the next breath to come, do not rush into the next breath	Allow the expiratory pause to lengthen, if comfortable to do so, to further slow respiratory rate and promote relaxation.

push them onwards as this will increase tension and frustration. Some patients, especially those with more severe disease, may not achieve all steps and may never get beyond step 2.

Step 1

The initial step focuses on relaxation of the breathing accessory muscles as well as relaxation of the mind and body. The breathing accessory muscles maybe particularly tense from daily use. Remember these not only include the inspiratory accessory muscles around the neck, shoulders and upper chest but also the expiratory accessory muscles around the abdomen. Any tight clothing or belts should be loosened. General relaxation techniques may be of benefit to patients who struggle at this step. The patient should nose breathe, if able and comfortable.

Step 2

This step is about noticing the abdominal movement with each breath but not try to change it. The patient is not forcing this movement through effort, they are just relaxing their breathing accessory muscles, which includes their abdominal muscles, and feeling the tummy rise and fall as they breathe.

Step 3

Once the patient is comfortable with feeling the abdominal movement you may like to then focus on how the diaphragm is used. Inspiration is active but only take in the air that is needed, no more. Ensure the patient understands we are not looking for a big movement at the tummy, it should be very subtle, just float the air in. Remind the patient that the diaphragm only moves down 1 cm during relaxed breathing at rest.

The out breath should be as passive as possible, don't waste extra energy, just relax and let go. Remind the patient that it is the elastic recoil of the lung and chest wall that creates expiration, no effort required, it will happen by its self. In severe obstructive lung disease (COPD/emphysema) expiratory accessory muscles of the abdomen may be required on expiration but the aim is to reduce to their activity to a comfortable minimum.

The expiration phase is important to allow breathing muscles to return to their resting length and for the inhaled tidal volume to be fully exhaled otherwise breath stacking and dynamic hyperinflation will result. Remember expiration time may also be longer than the 1:1.5–2 ratio in obstructive airways disease.

It is sometimes not helpful to deliberately lengthen exhalation in those with restrictive lung disease, such as pulmonary fibrosis or those with lung cancer, as this may cause discomfort and coughing due to airway collapse or compression at lower lung volumes.

Step 4

When a person's breathing is very relaxed there may be a short pause after expiration. Some patients may be able to notice this pause and then relax into it, allowing it to lengthen. Patients with more severe disease may not be able to achieve this. Some may find it uncomfortable, causing them to tense and upset their breathing pattern, so do not force it. Allow it to happen if it is comfortable.

Breathing Control vs Breathing Pattern Re-education

Some may argue that this in depth way of teaching Breathing Control goes beyond the definition of Breathing Control and moves into the realms of breathing pattern re-education, especially steps 3–5. However relaxing and lengthening the out breath and finding and resting in the expiratory pause help to slow respiratory rate and may reduce hyperventilation and hyperinflation, therefore helping to ease breathlessness.

Breathing Control and breathing pattern re-education both have the aim of achieving efficient breathing and therefore there will be some blurring of the boundaries. The BTS/ACPRC (2009) states that Breathing Control is "Normal tidal breathing encouraging relaxation of the upper chest and shoulders" The word 'normal' could also imply a normal breathing pattern as well as normal volume and therefore it appears appropriate to consider the pattern of breathing when teaching Breathing Control.

Some breathless patients with chronic heart or lung pathologies may have developed breathing pattern disorders not driven by their pathology but by 'bad habits' due to long term stress, anxiety or hyper-vigilance of breathing.

> Hyper-vigilance of breathing may cause patients to attribute unpleasant symptoms to pathology when in fact they may be due to hyperventilation, poor breathing pattern or inefficient breathing muscle use.

Improving breathing efficiency may help patients recognise what symptoms are pathology based and what can be changed through improved breathing.

Patients are encouraged to practice Breathing Control at rest when not breathless so that they are familiar with it in times of need. In breathing pattern retaining usually 1–2, 10 min sessions a day is recommended with regular breathing 'checks' during the day initiated by a frequent task such as boiling the kettle, opening a cupboard etc. Sometimes patients put a visual reminder i.e. sticker dot in places they frequent throughout the day. It is important patients do not become obsessive about their breathing and once 'checked' it should be forgotten (Bradley 2011).

This regular practice in its self is an opportunity to improve a patient's breathing pattern and efficiency of their breathing in general day to day life. It is therefore an opportunity not to be missed. Improving breathing pattern efficiency is a valuable part of the breathlessness management package. Some patients may not require much breathing pattern re-education while for others it may be a significant part of their management.

If the patient appears to show an abnormal breathing pattern or hyperventilation on exercise testing that cannot be attributed to pathology and that is not improved by teaching Breathing Control using the stages above then a review by Respiratory Physiotherapist with an interest in breathing pattern disorders (sometimes known as disordered breathing or chronic hyperventilation syndrome) is indicated.

Signs that may indicate a breathing pattern disorder in those with chronic heart or lung pathology

- Frequent sighs, yawns, sniffs, throat clearing coughs
- Habitual mouth breather, blocked nose
- Tense shoulders, upper chest breather
- Unnecessary accessory muscle use
- Large or variable tidal volumes, particularly at rest
- Fast or variable respiratory rate, particularly at rest
- Noisy breathing
- Hyperventilation just prior to activity, when speaking or during activity (shown on exercise testing)
- Variable quality of voice
- Disproportionate breathlessness compared with pathological impairment
- Symptoms of hyperventilation such as bilateral pins and needles in fingers or around mouth or light-headedness when breathless

Patients Who Find Breathing Control Difficult

Some patients struggle to relax their upper chest and feel the breathing movement at their abdomen. Often the harder they try to do the breathing technique correctly the more the breathing accessory muscles and upper chest movement come into play. Relaxation and 'trying less' is the key to success. Below are some ideas that may help patients who are struggling to master the technique.

Position and Posture

The affect of posture on breathing pattern and muscles use should not be underestimated. The most common postures to learn Breathing Control in is supported sitting in a chair or long sitting, with legs out straight in front, often with a pillow under the knees to improve comfort. If a patient is struggling with relaxation of the shoulders, upper chest and abdominal muscles it is worth trying a change of posture.

Consider a more supported position for an anxious patient or someone who finds it difficult to relax. Fully supported, with pillows under the arms and behind the head in long sitting or side lying with a pillow between the knees can be useful in such cases. Side lying is also a good position for a patient with a thoracic kyphosis or a large abdomen as it allows the abdominal contents to move forward out of the way of the diaphragm. The more supported and comfortable the position the easier it will be for the patient to relax their postural muscles of the abdominal wall, chest and shoulder muscles. The more their abdominal muscles relax the easier it will be for them to 'feel' the breathing movement of the diaphragm. Remember the head is heavy and therefore should be comfortably supported to encourage relaxation of the neck and shoulder muscles.

'Horse rider' position (sitting up-right on the edge or corner of a chair with legs apart and pelvis anteriorly tilted) helps some people to relax their upper chest and abdominal muscles.

Placing the hands behind the head or behind the back in sitting, long sitting or lying can help some people relax their shoulders and upper chest. Experiment with different positions to see which gives the best results.

Once Breathing Control has become familiar, the patient should practice using Breathing Control in other positions

This initial position is to help the patient learn the technique, however it may not necessarily be the best position to recover from breathlessness.

such as positions to ease breathlessness and functional positions for activities of daily living. They should also practice using Breathing Control during activity and exercise.

Abdominal Weight

In long sitting place a small weight, such as a small bean bag, and ask the patient to try to 'lift' the weight with their tummy as they breathe in. Children may like to 'lift the teddy' with their tummy. This may help patients initially 'feel' and see the breathing movement but should not be used long term as may encourage too much muscular effort and increased tidal volumes. Move to 'hand on tummy' as soon as able and ensure tidal volumes are appropriate.

Increased Tidal Volumes

Ask the patient exaggerate the breathing movement by taking deeper breaths in order to either feel the movement with their hands or to lift the abdominal weight. Once the patient can feel the abdominal breathing movement it is very important to then encourage the patient to relax their breathing and take in only the air they need with each breath. Ideally the abdominal movement should be slight and hardly notable at rest.

Two Hands: Upper Chest and Tummy

Start with the patient having one hand on their upper chest and their other hand on the tummy, between the umbilicus and the bottom ribs. Ensure shoulders are relaxed and elbows rest in at sides. As the patient breathes out ask them to focus on relaxing and 'letting go' or 'deflating' under the upper chest hand. On each in breath the patient should focus on 'feeling the tummy expand or inflate' and 'let the tummy hand rise' as they breathe in. Essentially the patient should try to reduce the chest movement under the 'top' hand while the bottom hand rises and falls with each breath. Once the patient feels they are 'breathing from their bottom hand' they can then move both hands to their tummy or just rest the 'upper chest' hand on their lap.

Two Hands: Tummy Only

The patient places both hands on their tummy with finger tips just touching. Ensure shoulders relaxed, elbows resting in at sides. As the patient breathes in they notice their finger tips separate, as they breathe out the finger tips touch again. Initially large breaths maybe required to notice this movement however once the patient has become familiar with this observation they should be encouraged to reduce the volume of the breaths to normal, to take just the air they need and no more, so the finger tips parting is very subtle.

Deflate the Upper Chest

Some patients struggle to lead with their diaphragm and tend to initiate the breath with their upper chest. Often they are over active in their upper chest muscles and hold tension and volume here. It may help for the clinician to place one or two hands on the upper chest and add some over pressure as the patient breathes out while asking the patient to 'deflate' the top of their chest. As the patient takes the next breath in encourage them to lead with their tummy and feel this movement with their own hand. The clinician maintains some over pressure to the upper chest as the patient breathes in to encourage them to 'keep the upper chest still'. Adjust over pressure to suit patient. Too strong a pressure maybe uncomfortable or cause panic. A soft pad between the clinician's hands and the patient's chest is recommended.

'Not Doing'

Some patients concentrate so much on 'achieving' abdominal movement that they forget the key to mastering the technique is relaxation of the mind, body and breathing accessory muscles. F. M. Alexander (founder of the Alexander Technique) taught the idea that if you stop doing the wrong thing then the right thing will happen by its self (Macdonald 1989). The patient may need to be reminded of this and the focus of the clinician's teaching should move away from encouraging abdominal movement to relaxation of mind, body and breathing accessory muscles.

In fact F. M. Alexander would go further as to say that efficient breathing cannot be taught and only through correct body alignment and muscle use will efficient breathing happen. Indeed we should also address muscle imbalances and poor posture that may hinder good breathing.

For patients with milder breathlessness who can comfortably lie flat without aggravating their symptoms, the Alexander semi supine position may help gain improved alignment, posture and muscle use, in particular around the neck and shoulders. In such a position efficient breathing may happen by its self and the patient just has to notice what it feels like. Suitable patients and interested clinicians may wish to take up Alexander lessons to explore this technique further (Fig. 5.3).

Relaxation Techniques

Breathing should be subconscious for it to be comfortable. Some people therefore become anxious and uncomfortable when they focus on their breathing. Other patients may just find it hard to relax generally. In such cases general whole

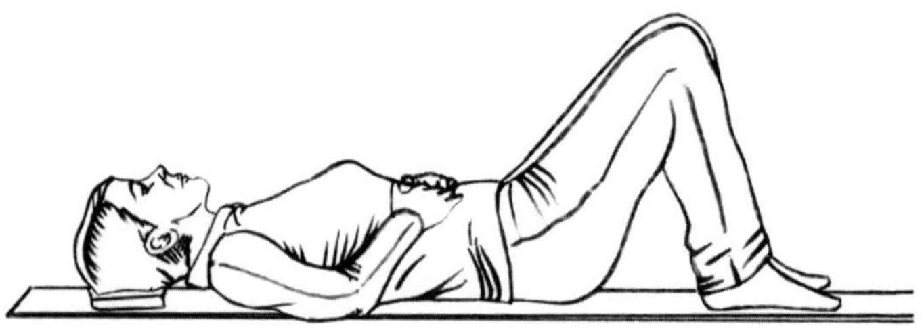

FIGURE 5.3 The Alexander semi supine position, © CBIS, 2013

body and mind relaxation should be the focus. Some patients, once more relaxed, may wish to return to learning formal Breathing Control. Others may continue general relaxation and efficient breathing may develop without formal breathing pattern re-education. Chap. 6: Anxiety Management provides further information on relaxation strategies.

No Observers

Some patients may just find it hard to relax when they are being watched. When teaching Breathing Control with others in the room, such as relatives or other members of staff, ask that everyone practices Breathing Control and to close their eyes if they wish. As the teacher you may like to close your eyes so the patient no longer believes you are watching them, you can later open your eyes to observe their breathing as you talk them through the technique. This ensures there are no 'observers' to make the patient feel uncomfortable. If others in the room are still a source of anxiety you may need to ask them to leave to take the patient to a different room.

Fear or Anxiety

Sometimes a patient's overriding fears regarding breathlessness, future deterioration in their condition, or breathlessness becoming uncontrolled and fear of death itself can override all attempts to improve relaxation and breathing pattern. The patient may not openly share their fears and may need support to talk about their concerns before progress can be made with learning breathing and relaxation techniques.

Observe Other Mammals

The patient may wish to observe their partner breathing when resting (if their partner has a good, relaxed pattern) or the way their cat or dog naturally breathes with their tummy when asleep. Obviously the patient should not try to copy the speed at which a smaller mammal breathes as the rate will be far too quick.

Keep It Simple

Do not expect to make your patient's breathing pattern 'perfect' in the first session. This may cause frustration for you and the patient. Keep things simple and allow the patient time to adjust. The patient's concentration may be very short at first. Once you feel they understand and are able to at least attempt a good breathing pattern then it is often best to review how they are doing in a few days or a week later. You may find they have made great progress while practicing alone, unpressured and unobserved. You can then progress technique if required.

Musculoskeletal

Thoracic, shoulder and neck stretches and mobilisation exercises should be considered for those with stiff joints and tight muscles from poor posture and chronic accessory muscle use.

Pain

Pain and discomfort increase muscular tension and may therefore pose a barrier to efficient breathing and will need to be addressed.

Alternatives to Breathing Control or Relaxation Techniques

Patients who find it difficult to focus on their breathing or on formal relaxation techniques may benefit from engaging an activity to improve their breathing pattern without direct focus. Such activities include Tai Chi, Yoga, Meditation, listening to music or engaging in a hobby or craft they find enjoyable and an escape from everyday worries. Tai Chi, Yoga or Meditation that involves deep, diaphragmatic breathing may not suit those with obstructive lung disease as may worsen hyperinflation and therefore increase breathlessness. Patients with milder forms of obstructive lung disease may be able to counter act the potential worsening hyperinflation caused by diaphragmatic breathing by pursed-lips breathing (discussed later in this chapter).

Severely Hyperinflated Lungs

Breathing Control may not be suitable for patients with severely hyperinflated lungs who have a flattened, inefficient diaphragm and therefore rely on their breathing accessory muscles even at rest. In such severe cases trying to teach patients to relax their breathing accessory muscles and breathe from 'their tummy' maybe futile and cause frustration to patient and clinician. Breathing techniques for hyperinflated lungs are discussed later in this chapter.

Case Study: Breathing Control and Breathlessness
Mrs Jennings, a 62 year old lady with lung cancer was referred to CBIS by her GP. Mrs Jennings said she liked being busy and became easily stressed. She sometimes felt a tightness in her chest and her voice became weak, especially after long conversations over the phone.

At rest Mrs Jennings was very tense in her upper chest and shoulders. She upper chest breathed in short, sharp breaths. Her breathing pattern worsened when she spoke about things that upset her. She complained of generalised aching at the back of her neck and across the back of her shoulders. On getting up from the chair she started hyperventilating even before moving.

She had discussed all these symptoms with her oncologist who had investigated and concluded they were linked to stress however Mrs Jennings was still worried that it was the cancer that was causing them.

Treatment
Five sessions with CBIS clinicians with follow up phone calls. Treatment included:

- Discussing Mrs Jennings fears regarding diagnosis and prognosis as well as her fears regarding her symptoms.
- Discussing 'good' and 'bad' breathing habits and how stress and muscle tension may cause a change in breathing i.e. when on the phone Mrs Jennings was often talking about her cancer and fears and that's when she lost her voice.
- Discussed symptoms of hyperventilation and how changes in breathing and muscle tension around the neck and upper chest can cause changes to the voice.
- She found Breathing Control very difficult to master so we started with general relaxation techniques, gentle mobilising exercises for shoulders and upper chest and posture correction.
- Returned to Breathing Control and practiced in side lying to aid relaxation as she was too tense in sitting.
- Mrs Jennings tried 'too hard' to achieve Breathing Control so we talked of other things while her had

was on her tummy. When she relaxed and started naturally tummy breathing I pointed out how calm and relaxed her breathing had become and how beautifully she was breathing from her tummy. I asked her to remember this feeling and way of breathing and try to practice it in side lying each day.

- Eventually she progressed to using Breathing Control when sitting, standing and moving.
- Once Breathing Control was mastered we practice reading aloud the alphabet and numbers at first and then simple children's books and poetry. Mrs Jennings was encouraged to keep her shoulders and upper chest relaxed, her voice calm and measured, breathe from her tummy and take regular breaths at natural pauses at punctuation marks.
- Drew attention to hyperventilation prior to movement and practiced keeping breathing calm and from the tummy with shoulders and upper chest relaxed while going from lie to sit to stand and then walking, with pauses to control breathing as required.

Outcome

Aches and discomfort have resolved. Posture improved, shoulders and upper chest relaxed. No longer looses voice or becomes tight chested during phone calls. No longer hyperventilates prior and during activity. Mrs Jennings was much calmer in general and continues to take time out daily for relaxation. She was no longer worried that the symptoms were caused by her cancer.

Visual Aids to Memory

Regular practice of Breathing Control at rest allows patients to become familiar with making their breathing as relaxed and efficient as possible. However during a time of breathlessness

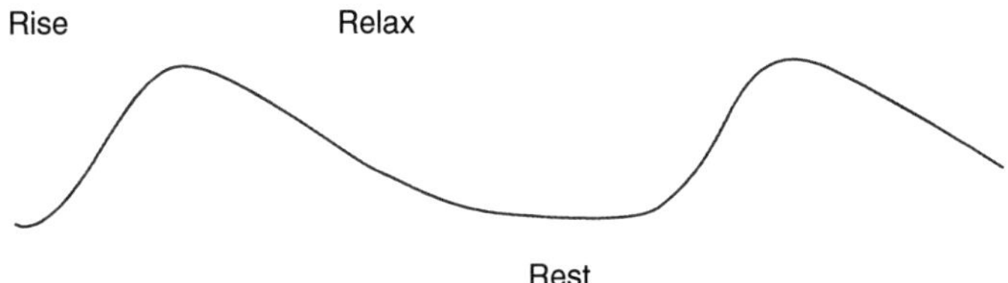

FIGURE 5.4 The Rise, Relax and Rest wave of Breathing Control © CBIS, 2013

it can be difficult to remember what to do therefore aids to memory may help remind patients of the essence of Breathing Control.

The 3 R's

Repeating the 3 R's : **R**ise, **R**elax, **R**est in the mind as they feel the tummy movement with their hand can be both relaxing and aid memory of the Breathing Control technique.

The 3 R's of Breathing Control (Relaxed Tummy Breathing)

- **R**ise: Tummy rises as you breathe in.
- **R**elax: Relax the tummy, relax the breath out.
- **R**est: Don't rush into the next breath, wait for it to come.

Waves

It may be helpful to visualise the image of a wave while practicing or using Breathing Control (Fig. 5.4). Breaths can be visualised as waves on a beach, some waves maybe bigger than others and some waves maybe closer together but they still keep coming at their own gentle pace. Remember expiration is passive therefore takes a little longer than the inspiration.

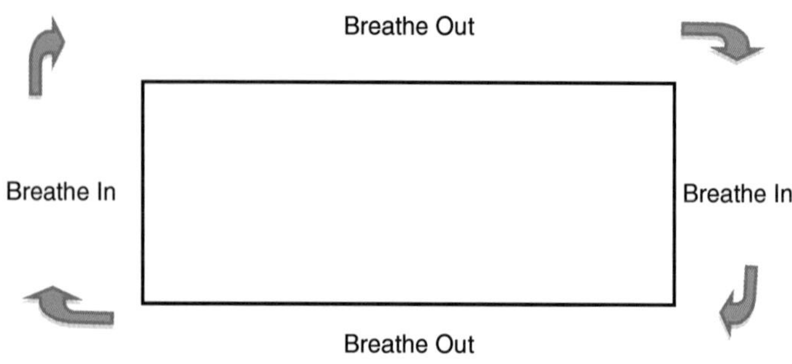

FIGURE 5.5 Breathing rectangle © CBIS, 2013

Breathing Rectangle

Wherever you are you can usually see a rectangle somewhere; a book, a window, a door, a picture, a television, a computer screen, to name just a few. While focusing on Breathing Control it may help to follow the edge of a rectangle with the eyes to pace and slow the breathing. To 'breathe around a rectangle' the patient breathes in while looking along the shorter side, then breathes out while following the longer side (Fig. 5.5). Gradually slowing down the pace at which their eyes move around the rectangle will help slow their breathing.

Patients may find it useful to have a drawing of a rectangle on their personal plans or personal breathlessness management 'flash cards'. Patients with obstructive airways disease may require a longer, thinner rectangle as their expiration is often prolonged due to the obstructive nature of their condition. Additionally deliberately prolonging the out breath may allow more time for exhalation and help to reduce dynamic hyperinflation in such patients, especially if combined with pursed-lips breathing.

Case Study: Newly Diagnosed COPD
Mr Robertson, is a 44 year old gentleman who was diagnosed with mild COPD the previous year during hospital admission for pneumonia. Following this he took

4 months off work as a builder and returned part time. Mr Robertson was referred to CBIS from respiratory clinic with disproportionate breathlessness on exertion. Cardiopulmonary testing that showed hyperventilation during exercise and as well as some reduced fitness.

When exerting himself Mr Robertson feels he needs to get more air into his lungs "I can't get a full lung of air" and then he panics, making the problem worse. He is concerned about exercise and becoming breathless at work during heavy work as builder "Is it harmful?" he asks. His partner is also concerned. Mr Robertson still smokes, he has tried the local stop smoking service before but failed to quit. He does not want to waste their time.

During the initial assessment Mr Robertson clears his throat a lot when talking. He is an upper chest mouth breather with tense shoulders and a variable tidal volume. He has very good oxygen saturations at rest and does not desaturate on exercise.

Treatment

Three home visits with the CBIS physiotherapist and follow up phone calls. Treatment included:

- Discussing fears related to diagnosis, prognosis and breathlessness.
- Anxiety and breathlessness link.
- Showed patient that he does not desaturate on exercise.
- 'Normal' breathing vs hyperventilation discussed.
- Discussed hyperinflation and how this may make the chest feel tight and unable to take a deep breath.
- Importance of the out breathe to release the air and to not focus deliberately taking large breaths in.
- Importance of nose breathing, Buteyko nose clearing exercises (+).
- Breathing Control and breathing pattern re-education at rest and on exertion.

- Hand held fan.
- Positions of ease.
- Importance of exercise explained and how it may help with breathlessness management.
- Game console jogging programme.
- Referred to GP gym scheme.
- Discussion of importance of quitting smoking and that many attempts may be required.
- Stop smoking service re-referral accepted.
- Advised on work and breathlessness management: regular breaks, avoid prolonged upper limb work above head, repeated bending or flexed positions. Advised on use of paced breathing and 'blow as you go' when at work, in addition to Breathing Control.

Outcomes

Date of visit	SOB at rest	SOB on exertion*	Anxiety at rest	Anxiety on exertion*
18th Nov (1st visit)	1	6	1	7
6th Jan (final visit)	0.5	2	0	0

SOB (shortness of breath) & anxiety measured using the modified Borg score (*Exertion is defined as walking ¼ mile at own steady pace).

Mr. Robertson's nose is clear and can nose breathe at rest and during exercise. He has a relaxed abdominal breathing pattern at rest, relaxed shoulders, no throat clearing. He uses Breathing Control when in van at work during breaks and during work activity and when exercising, along with other breathing techniques taught. He has begun GP gym scheme and uses games console jogging program daily. He is engaging with Camquit and has stuck to quit date. Long term goal: Would like to return to full time work. He is considering changing job to active job but with less heavy lifting.

This case study shows how the fear of breathlessness being harmful and poor breathing patterns can lead to decreased fitness and ability to work even in young, newly diagnosed mild COPD, highlighting the importance of early intervention.

(+) Brindley et al. (2012)

Dynamic Hyperinflation

"*I just can't get my breath in, my chest feels so tight, I don't know where the next breath is coming from.*"- A gentleman with COPD.

There is a strong correlation between exertional dyspnoea, end-expiratory lung volume & inspiratory effort to volume displacement. (O'Donnell 2006)

Hyperinflation is a significant causative factor for breathlessness in those with obstructive airways disease such as COPD, emphysema and asthma. In COPD and emphysema dynamic hyperinflation is usually additional to static hyperinflation and occurs during episodes of increased ventilatory demand, such as when exercising. In severe obstructive airways disease dynamic hyperinflation may occur during arm function alone (Marin et al. 2001).

Adverse Effects of Hyperinflation

- Forces respiratory muscles to work at shortened lengths therefore reducing their force generation capacity, shortening their range and the time available for force generation.

- Lung compliance reduces (becomes stiffer) as the lungs near their maximum stretch, the inward elastic recoil of the lungs is stronger, increasing work of breathing.
- The more hyperinflated the lungs are, the harder the work of breathing and the more breathless a person feels.

Dynamic hyperinflation can occur in healthy athletes when exercising due to reduced exhalation length causing breath stacking as breathing becomes more rapid during intense exercise (Folinsbee et al. 1983). In a similar way dynamic hyperinflation may occur in patients who do not have a pathology that predisposes them to hyperinflation. A patient who is very breathless, perhaps due to anxiety or panic, may breathe so rapidly that they do not allow adequate time for exhalation and therefore cause dynamic hyperinflation and a feeling of 'tight chest' and 'unable to breathe deeply' which may exacerbate their panic and anxiety.

The more hyperinflated the lungs are the smaller the potential tidal volume available to the patient, therefore the less 'room to breathe'. Patients often describe not being able 'to get enough air', 'I can't catch my breath', 'I can't get the air in' and 'I don't know where the next breath is coming from'. They may panic and try to take deeper breaths which will only worsen the dynamic hyperinflation. Hyperinflation also puts the breathing muscles, particularly the diaphragm, at a mechanical disadvantage, reducing their force generating capacity and therefore reducing their potential to aid ventilation.

If hyperinflation is a significant factor in a patient's breathlessness then this should be explained to the patient. Having an understanding of a physical reason for breathlessness may remove some of the fear and the patient's focus on the common miss conception that 'breathlessness must mean my oxygen levels are low'.

The clinician should then explain and teach techniques that may help them when breathless to reduce hyperinflation, such as pursed-lips breathing and focusing on longer out breaths, to 'let the old air out to create space for the next breath in'. If possible, patients should avoid deliberately taking in large breaths when breathless as this can be counterproductive.

Bronchodilators have been shown to reduce hyperinflation at rest (Newton et al. 2002) and during exercise in those with moderate to severe COPD (Belman et al. 1996). Some patients with COPD who are prescribed a short acting bronchodilator to be taken as required (PRN) may find using this inhaler prior to exercise may reduce dynamic hyperinflation and therefore the intensity of breathlessness they experience.

Pursed-Lips Breathing

"*Creating room to breathe*"

> Pursed-lips breathing has been defined as "The generation of positive pressure within the airways by expiration against partially closed lips" (BTS/ACPRC 2009, p.i50).

Pursed-lips breathing (PLB) can be described to patients as if they were pursing their lips as if about to blow a kiss or to preparing to whistle. PLB has also been described as 'sniff the rose, flicker the candle'. Exhalation length when PLB has been described as twice to four times the length of inspiration or breathe out for as long as you can, however forceful exhalation should be avoided.

PLB slows and prolongs the out breath and can create an average expiratory pressure of 5 cm H_2O at the mouth (Van der Schans et al. 1995). This expiratory pressure inhibits airway collapse, improving expiratory flow and therefore reducing dynamic hyperinflation, which allows for an improvement in tidal volume during exercise (Bianchi et al. 2007). This back pressure (positive end expiratory pressure) maybe described to patients as if they are using their thumb to partially obstruct the end of a hosepipe to spray water when watering the garden. This back pressure holds the airways open and allows the 'old' air to escape therefore creating space for the next breath in, thus 'creating room to breathe'.

Research Evidence

PLB has the strongest research based of all the breathing techniques used in breathlessness management. PLB is recommended for the management of breathlessness in those with COPD (BTS/ACPRC 2009).

The Potential Benefits of PLB

- Reduce respiratory rate by nearly 7 breaths per minute
- Increase tidal volume by 500 mL
- Improve oxygen saturations by 2.5 %

Leading to:

- Improved recovery rate from exertional breathlessness
- Improved functional performance

Conclusions of a systematic review of the evidence by Roberts et al. (2009)

Instinctive PLB

"*I've told him to stop puffing with his mouth, he doesn't breathe right*"- Wife of a patient with COPD

PLB may reduce breathlessness during activity and speed recovery from breathlessness after exertion. It is often adopted instinctively by people with severe COPD. Spahija et al. (2010) found that patients who instinctively PLB had greater hypercapnia, lower exercise tolerance, lower diffusion capacity, more hyperinflated lungs and greater resting breathlessness than those who did not PLB.

If a patient instinctively PLB then it is worth educating the patient and their carers as to why PLB is beneficial. Not only does this help the patient to gain confidence in their ability to manage their breathlessness but it may also prevent their carers 'nagging' their loved one to 'breathe correctly'. Grunting when very breathless works in a similar way to PLB but the positive end expiratory pressure is created by the vocal cords.

Can PLB Be Taught?

Unfortunately research on PLB has been confounded over the years by researcher's different interpretation of the technique as well as subject selection, with subjects having mixture of mild to severe COPD in one cohort giving mixed results as to the benefit of PLB. This has led to the debate regarding whether PLB can be taught and if so, do patients voluntarily continue its use for daily breathlessness management.

Patients with mild to moderate airflow obstruction and therefore without significant hyperinflation as a cause for their breathlessness have found PLB may increase their work of breathing, without an improvement in their breathlessness or tidal volume (Spahija et al. 2005). PLB therefore does not help all patients with obstructive airways disease. If PLB is to be taught then patient selection is important. Bianchi et al. (2007) found that subjects with more severe COPD (average FEV_1 of 38 %) gained the most benefit from PLB.

Patients who adopt PLB instinctively often gain the greatest benefits. However Nield et al. (2007) found that short term benefits of PLB translated to longer term improvements in quality of life at 3 months follow up when PLB was taught to subjects who did not PLB instinctively.

Explaining PLB to Patients and Carers
"When someone has chronic obstructive lung disease, due to changes in the airways, air tends to get trapped in the lungs, especially when breathless. As you breathe

in the lungs expand and the air comes in. As you breathe out the airways may flop closed causing air to become trapped in the lungs. Pursed lips breathing creates a back pressure in the airways, like putting your thumb over the end of a hose pipe when spraying water on the garden. This back pressure holds the airways open as you breathe out and allows the air to escape from the lungs. It also lengthens the out breath allowing more time for the air to leave the lungs, therefore creating room for the next breathe in. Essentially letting the old air out to create room to breathe".

Teaching PLB

When teaching PLB the aim is to narrow the lips enough to gain benefit but not so much that the increased work of breathing outweighs the benefit. Roberts et al. (2009) suggested that biofeedback from pulse oximeter may aid in teaching PLB to those who do not PLB distinctively. While PLB at rest the patient should aim to improve their oxygen saturation while the clinician looks for a fall respiratory rate. If these are observed then this indicates the patient may benefit from PLB. The patient should then practice PLB at rest, during activities that make them breathless and to speed their recovery when they become breathless. After a 4-week trial, if no benefits have been seen, then PLB is discontinued.

PLB can be an 'add on' to other breathing techniques. The clinician may suggest a patient adds PLB to expiration when using Breathing Control or Recovery Breathing.

Recovery Breathing: The 3 F's

"*I hadn't realised that the more you let your breath out, the more relaxed you become*" – A lady with COPD.

"She told me that it is best to get your breath out because your breath will always go in; and not to take deep breaths. Yeah and its really helped."- A gentleman with COPD.

Recovery Breathing – 'The 3 Fs'

Fan
Forward lean
Focus on……
………… long breaths out*
………… relaxing the breath out*
(*Select according to pathology)

When very breathless and panicky some patients feel they need to breathe 'in, in, in…' with the misconception to 'get more oxygen' and therefore focus on taking in as much air as possible. This panicky, rapid breathing pattern may reduce expiratory time therefore not allowing lungs to empty fully and cause breath stacking, leading to dynamic hyperinflation. The patient may feel their chest is more and more tight and restricted as they do this, no matter what their pathology.

Patients can be so focused on filling their lungs, to 'get more oxygen' that they forget that there is only one way into the lungs and only one way out. Whatever amount of air they take in they must also breathe out, otherwise there will be with no space for the next breath.

Deliberately lengthening the out breath may help reduce dynamic hyperinflation and therefore create 'room to breathe'. It may also help to tell the patient not to worry about the in breath, it will take care of its self. Very breathless or panicking patients may find it difficult to deliberately slow their breathing rate. By focusing on lengthening or relaxing the out breath, the rate of breathing should naturally slow down without deliberate focus (Fig. 5.6).

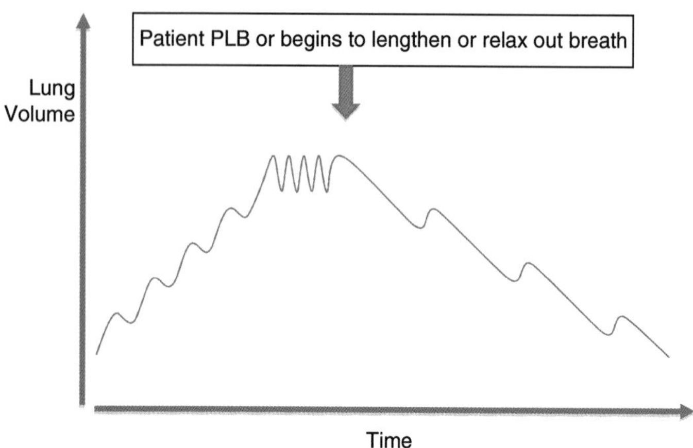

FIGURE 5.6 The effect of PLB or lengthening/relaxing the out breath on breath stacking and hyperinflation PLB © CBIS, 2013

The concept of the 3 Fs of Recovery Breathing, was developed by the Cambridge Breathlessness Intervention Service to help reduce dynamic hyperinflation, and therefore ease breathing, in situations of severe breathless or panic. Some institutions have renamed the technique 'rescue breathing' to match the 'rescue' packs of medication of exacerbations.

Explaining Recovery Breathing to Patients and Carers
"When someone is very breathless or panicky they may focus on taking in as much air as possible to try to improve their breathing. There is only one way in and out of the lungs. Whatever amount of air is taken in must also come out. By focusing on breathing in, in, in... the lungs can fill up like two balloons until there is little space for the next breath. This is often when people feel tight chested and that they 'can't get my breath'. By focusing on long out breaths you let the old air out and create room for the next breath in, creating room to breathe".

When to Use Recovery Breathing

A Patient Unfamiliar with Breathing Control

Breathing Control often takes practice to master before it can be used effectively in situations of severe breathlessness. Patients with milder breathlessness may be able to learn Breathing Control 'on the spot' however most patients require careful teaching and practice of Breathing Control when not breathless. Recovery Breathing maybe more easily taught 'on the spot' than Breathing Control to help calm a patient who is very breathless or panicky.

Patients with Severely Hyperinflated Lungs

"*They told me to breathe with my tummy but I just can't, why don't they understand, it's so frustrating*"- Gentleman with severe emphysema

Patients with severely hyperinflated lungs from COPD or emphysema have flattened and inefficient diaphragms. Such patients may therefore rely on their respiratory accessory muscles even at rest. Teaching Breathing Control by focusing on diaphragm use and relaxation of accessory muscles can be futile and may end in frustration for both the clinician and patient, especially in situations where the patient's breathlessness is exacerbated by activity. Recovery Breathing may be beneficial to aid recovery from exertional breathlessness in such patients. This technique maybe enhanced by pursed-lips breathing during exhalation.

Extreme Breathlessness and Panic

Patients with breathlessness of any pathology may find Recovery Breathing useful in situations of extreme breathlessness or panic if they find, for whatever reason, they are unable to use Breathing Control effectively.

Modifying Recovery Breathing

Lengthening the out breath does not suit every pathology therefore Recovery Breathing should be modified depending on the underlying condition and whether hyperinflation is a significant causative factor for breathlessness.

Modifying the Focus of the Out Breath

- **Hyperinflating Pathologies** (i.e. COPD, emphysema, asthma): Focus on **long** out breaths +/– pursed-lip breathing. Lengthening the exhalation time, with or without the positive end expiratory pressure of pursed-lips breathing may help to reduce dynamic hyperinflation. Suggest the patient 'deflates' as they breathe out. Perhaps focus this deflation on the upper chest by placing your hand here as you ask them to 'deflate'.
- **Non-hyperinflating Pathologies** (i.e. lung cancer, heart failure, restrictive lung disease such as pulmonary fibrosis): Focus on **relaxing** the out breath. Patients with restrictive lung conditions may feel panicky and more breathless if they lengthen the out breath. Patients with lung cancer sometime begin to cough when lengthening the out breath, perhaps due to the pressure of tumours closing the airways at lower lung volumes.
- **Hyperventilation or Panic**: Either **lengthen or relax** the out breath. If you suspect non-pathological hyperinflation then encourage 'deflation' by lengthening the out breath. Sometimes lengthening the out breath aids relaxation and release of tension especially if they let their shoulders and upper chest 'drop and flop' with the out breath. However some patients may force the out breath and then feel air hunger. In such cases just relax the out breath along with shoulder and upper chest relaxation.

When encouraging patients to **lengthen** or **relax** the out breath it may help to suggest they imagine a 'wave' of relaxation, calm, peace or tranquillity flowing down from head to toes as they relax the out breath.

"Blow as You Go!"

Encouraging patients to "Blow as you go!"; that is to breathe out on effort, stretching or bending, may reduce breathlessness by improving respiratory mechanics during activity (BTS/ACPRC 2009). It is therefore preferable to the instinctive breath holding that patients sometimes do in such circumstances

Paced Breathing

"Breathing to a rhythm- for example in time with walking or stairs, to maintain control of breathing and thereby reduce dyspnoea" (BTS/ACPRC 2009 p.i50)

Some patients may rush activities, such as climbing the stairs, as they wrongly believe that if they 'get there quicker' they will become less breathless, when in fact the opposite is true. Paced Breathing can help a patient to slow down while keeping their breathing pattern efficient and controlled. An example of paced breathing is to breathe in on one step, breathe out on the next step when climbing the stairs. For more severe breathlessness the patient may need to pause on each step and take a 'normal sized' breath in and out before proceeding to the next step.

If a patient tends to rush when walking then suggest they practice breathing in for one step, out for two steps as they walk. The out breath takes more steps as expiration is always longer than inspiration. Patients may need to 'experiment' to find their own comfortable rhythm. This style of walking needs to be practised regularly for patients to become familiar and comfortable with the technique. This practice in its self may become a relaxing form of 'mindful or meditative walking'. In obstructive lung disease an increased number of steps may be needed to prolong the out breath to allow adequate time for exhalation to help avoid breath stacking and reduce dynamic hyperinflation.

It is not easy to slow down walking or climbing stairs. It may help to convince a patient by timing how long it takes them to 'rush' up stairs and then recover their breathing compared to pacing their breathing as they climb the stairs and then not needing a prolonged recovery time.

Case Study: Incident of Severe Breathlessness

Mrs Jacob, a 55 year old lady with moderate to severe COPD. She was normally not anxious about breathlessness as had 'become use to it over time' but had one bad experience while on holiday this year when she was walking back to the villa and became very breathless and panicky, she could not 'get the air in' and thought she 'was not going to make it'. Husband also found this experience very stressful.

Treatment

Two visits by CBIS physiotherapist and follow up phone calls. Treatment included:

- Discussed severe breathlessness incident with patient and husband. What happened, what was going through their minds, what did they find helped, is there anything they would do differently with hind sight?
- Discussed hyperinflation causing breathlessness in COPD and how this can cause the feeling of unable to 'get the air in'.

- Gave hand held fan and taught Recovery Breathing combined with pursed-lips breathing, to both patient and husband, as a strategy to manage a similar incident of breathlessness should it arise again in the future.
- Gave a personal laminated 'flash card' of the 3 Fs of Recovery breathing and pictures of forward lean positions.
- Discussed paced breathing and planning activities so that maybe able to avoid situation in the future.
- Also reviewed breathing pattern at rest and during exertion and made this as efficient as possible.

Outcome

Patient and husband felt confident that they could manage a similar situation in the future. They planned activities better, looking for opportunities to rest if required and ensured plenty of time to pace themselves so no need to rush. Mrs Jacob kept her hand held fan with her at all times, with the laminated card.

Nose vs Mouth Breathing

The nose is widely recognised as the 'air conditioning' system for the lungs. It warms, filters, humidifies and through nitric oxide, which is antimicrobial, cleanses the air. Nitric oxide is also a bronchodilator and vasodilator and therefore may have a role in ventilation and perfusion matching within the lungs. Nose breathing may also help deter hyperventilation.

Breathless patients often revert to mouth breathing as their work of breathing increases as the mouth is a larger orifice and therefore produces less resistance to air flow. This may lead some patients habitually mouth breathe unnecessarily at rest when they are not breathless. It is important to challenge this and encourage the patient to breathe through the nose at rest, if possible. This may take some getting used to and may require perseverance. Of course, some patients maybe significantly breathless at rest or have such a severe condition that they are unable to nose breathe at rest.

When using a breathing technique to ease breathlessness patients may find it useful to move from **mouth-mouth** breathing (in and out through mouth) to **nose-mouth** breathing (in through nose, out through mouth) to **nose-nose** breathing (in and out through nose) as their breathing eases.

Nose-mouth breathing (in through nose, out through mouth) may particularly help those with dynamic hyperinflation as it reduces inspiratory flow while promoting expiratory flow. Some patients report nose : mouth breathing is calming, it helps them to avoid 'gulping' in excess air. Some breathless patients actually find **nose-nose** breathing (in and out through nose) when using a breathing technique helps to calm their breathing and assists them to 'engage' with their diaphragm, encouraging abdominal movement.

All patients should aim to return to just nose breathing at rest, if possible. If the nose is blocked it may be worth trying some Buteyko nose clearing exercises (Brindley et al. 2012) or speaking to their GP about whether anything can be done to help clear the nose.

Flash Cards

It can be helpful to create a 'flash card' with a brief reminder of the breathing technique in the patient's own words if possible.

A flash card may include a picture of a position of ease, a positive affirmation such as 'breathlessness is not harmful, it will recover with rest', a rectangle or wave diagram as a visual aid and a reminder to use their fan (Fig. 5.7). The patient may

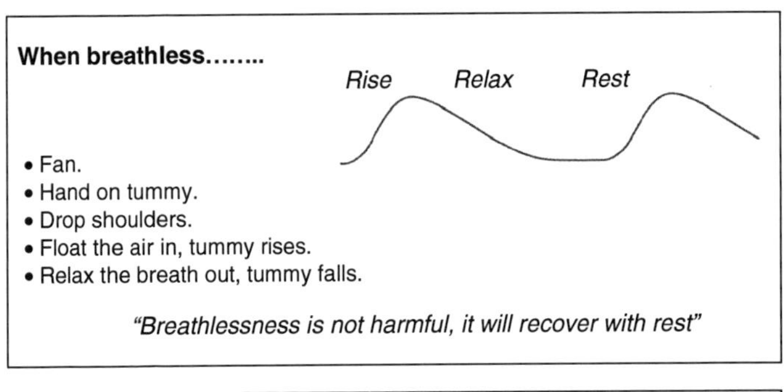

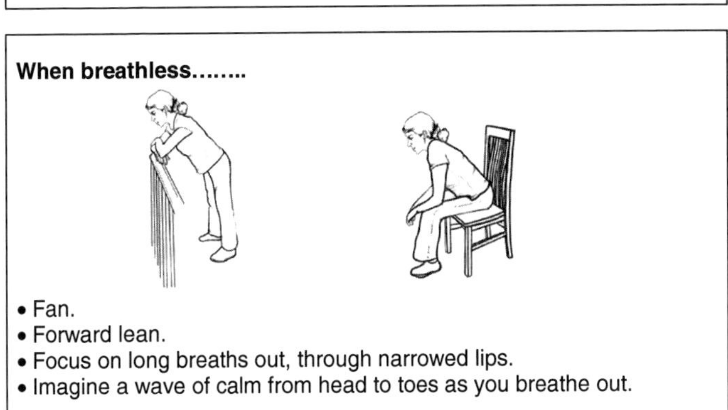

FIGURE 5.7 Two examples of flash cards, © CBIS, 2013

like to keep this card by their fan or on their bedside with their fan if night time breathlessness or panic is a problem. It is important to ensure the carer is familiar with breathing technique and other advice given. This may not only help the carer support the patient in times of need but also helps the carer to feel less anxious or helpless in such situations.

Summary

It can be very empowering for a patient to understand and master a breathing technique suited to their needs. Breathing techniques require no equipment and can be used anywhere and at anytime. Mastering a breathing technique can improve

TABLE 5.3 Comparison of possible technique selection to suit patient

A patient with lung cancer with anxiety and poor breathing pattern	A patient with severe COPD with severely hyperinflated lungs and accessory muscle use at rest
Relaxation techniques and explain anxiety-breathlessness link	Recovery breathing with pursed-lips breathing and long breaths out during activity and to recover from breathlessness
Nose breathing	Paced breathing and 'blow as you go'
Breathing Control at rest, during activity and to recover from breathlessness	Positions to ease breathlessness, may prefer positions with less flexion at abdomen to avoid 'fixing' diaphragm between abdominal contents and hyperinflated lungs
Breathing pattern re-education	
Positions of ease encouraging relaxation of upper chest and shoulders i.e. passive upper limb fixing	
May suit both patients	
Fan	
Encourage wave of relaxation from head to toe as breathe out	
Posture, mobilisation exercise and stretches	

the patient's confidence in their ability to manage their own breathlessness. Using a breathing technique provides a positive focus during an episode of breathlessness and may therefore help avoid frightening thoughts.

When selecting and teaching a breathing technique it is not 'one size fits all' (Table 5.3). Consider the patient's intuitive strategies and try to build on these, take into account the pathology and mechanics causing the breathlessness as well as the severity of the disease. Modify and combine breathing techniques to suit the patient and do not forget to combine breathing techniques with positions of ease, positive affirmations and the fan or other form of facial cooling.

Key Points

- Select the breathing technique to suit the patient, it's not 'one size fits all'.
- Consider combining the breathing technique with the fan, position of ease and positive affirmations.
- Pursed-lips breathing may be added to other breathing techniques such as Breathing Control, Recovery Breathing, Paced Breathing and 'Blow as you go'.
- Provide patient with a personal, simple 'flash card' as a reminder of the breathing technique, positions of ease, positive affirmations and to use fan.

References

Bradley D. Hyperventilation syndrome breathing pattern disorders and how to overcome them. London: Kyle Books; 2011.

Bianchi R, Gigliotti F, Romagnoli I, Lanini B, Castella C, Binazzi B, et al. Patterns of chest wall kinematics during volitional pursed-lip breathing in COPD at rest. Respir Med. 2007;101(7):1412–8.

Belman MJ, Botnick WC, Shin JW. Inhaled bronchodilators reduce dynamic hyperinflation during exercise in patients with chronic obstructive pulmonary disease. Am J Respir Crit Care Med. 1996;153(3):967–75.

Brindley J, Olive J, Godfrey K, Austin G, Shampan L . Buteyko breathing technique: teacher training manual. 3rd ed. Chipping Ongar. The Buteyko Breathing Association; 2012.

British Thoracic Society & Association of Chartered Physiotherapists in Respiratory Care (BTS/ACPRC). Guidelines for the physiotherapy management of the adult, medical, spontaneously breathing patient. Thorax. 2009;64(Supplement I):i1–51.

Folinsbee LJ, Wallace ES, Bedi JF, Horvath SM. Exercise respiratory pattern in elite cyclists and sedentary subjects. Med Sci Sports Exerc. 1983;15(6):503–9.

Gosselink RA, Wagnenaar RC, Rijswijki H, et al. Diaphragmatic breathing reduces the efficiency of breathing in patients with chronic obstructive pulmonary disease. Am J Respir Crit Care Med. 1995;151:1136–42.

Macdonald P. The Alexander technique as I see it. Brighton: Rahula Books; 1989.

Marin JM, Carrizo SJ, Gascon M, Sanchez A, Gallego B, Celli BR. Inspiratory capacity, dynamic hyperinflation, breathlessness and exercise performance during the 6-minute-walk test in chronic obstructive pulmonary disease. Am J Respir Crit Care Med. 2001; 162:1395–9.

Nield MA, Soo Hoo GW, Roper JM, Santiago S. Efficacy of pursed lips breathing: a breathing pattern retraining strategy for dyspnoea reduction. J Cardiopulm Rehabil Prev. 2007;27(4):237–44.

Newton MF, O'Donnell DE, Forkert L. Response of lung volumes to inhaled salbutamol in a large population of patients with severe hyperinflation. Chest. 2002;121(4):1042–50.

National Institute for Health and Care Excellence (NICE). Lung cancer: the diagnosis and treatment of lung cancer. CG 121. London: National Institute for Health and Care Excellence; 2011.

O'Donnell DE. Hyperinflation, dyspnoea and exercise tolerance in COPD. Proc Am Thorac Soc. 2006;3:180–4.

Roberts SE, Stern M, Schreuder FM, Watson T. The use of pursed lips breathing in stable chronic obstructive pulmonary disease: a systematic review of the evidence. Phys Ther Rev. 2009;14(4):240–6.

Spahija J, Marchie M, Ghezzo H, Grassino A. Factors discriminating spontaneous pursed-lips breathing use in patients with COPD. COPD. 2010;7(4):254–61.

Spahija J, de Marchie M, Grassino A. Effects of imposed pursed-lips breathing on respiratory mechanics and dyspnoea at rest and during exercise in COPD. Chest. 2005;128(2):640–50.

West JB. Respiratory physiology the essentials. 8th ed. Philadelphia: Lippincott Williams & Wilkins; 2008.

Van der Schans CP, De Jong W, Kort E, Wijkstra PJ, Koeter GH, Postma DS, et al. Mouth pressures during pursed lip breathing. Physiother Theory Pract. 1995;11:29–34.

Vitacca M, Clini E, Banchi L, et al. Acute effects of deep diaphragmatic breathing in COPD patients with chronic respiratory insufficiency. Eur Respir J. 1998;11:408–15.

Part III
Non-pharmacological Interventions – Thinking

Chapter 6
Anxiety Management

Evidence

The association between anxiety and breathlessness is well documented. Indeed some studies have been conducted which highlight the activation of the amygdala, part of the limbic system which plays a key role in the processing of emotions, in inducing breathlessness in healthy individuals, indicating this link (Banzett et al. 2000). There is no substantial evidence to recommend a definitive intervention for anxiety management for the breathless patient and much of the research to date calls for further, more robust investigation in to interventions which aim to reduce anxiety related to breathlessness. However, there is an increasing body of evidence to suggest that anxiety management techniques such as relaxation, mindfulness and cognitive behavioural therapy (CBT) can help with managing symptoms such as pain, stress and anxiety (Gustavsson and von Koch 2006; Kroner-Herwig 2009; Thompson 2009; Hunot et al. 2010). Booth et al. (2011) found that although anxiety management is frequently used with breathless patients, there is a need for definition and further research. Bauswein et al. (2008) also found insufficient data to analyse these interventions specifically for breathlessness. Studies are often small with limited

S. Booth et al., *Managing Breathlessness in Clinical Practice*,
DOI 10.1007/978-1-4471-4754-1_6,

numbers (Yorke et al. 2009) thus making it difficult to draw any conclusions from the research. However, complex interventions aimed to improve multiple symptoms, including breathlessness, such as pulmonary rehabilitation programmes or a multi-disciplinary team intervention for breathlessness, which incorporate a large element of anxiety management techniques such as relaxation, breathing control, challenging unhelpful thoughts and realistic goal setting, have strong evidence to support their effectiveness (Paz-Diaz et al. 2007).

Introduction

Establishing how a person actually feels about experiencing breathlessness is fundamental and provides an invaluable insight into the impact of this symptom on their lives. It is also important to ask carers and relatives how they feel when the person becomes breathless as this response can often influence subsequent actions, such as decisions to contact emergency services.

Patients will not often report directly that they feel "anxious" about their breathlessness. They may well describe associated emotions of panic, concern, worry, fear or immense frustration. When such sensations are evoked, this triggers the body's acute stress response also described as the "fight-or-flight-or-freeze" response. This physiological reaction occurs in response to a perceived harmful event or threat to survival, and in this case the perceived threat is breathlessness (Fig. 6.1). Explaining this response to patients and how it can influence breathlessness can go some way to reducing some of the manifestations of anxiety (such as sweating, needing to go to the toilet or palpitations) and can increase understanding as to why these occur. It can also help to reassure patients that there are some strategies and techniques that can help to control this response and, indeed, prevent it from happening altogether. Understanding why something

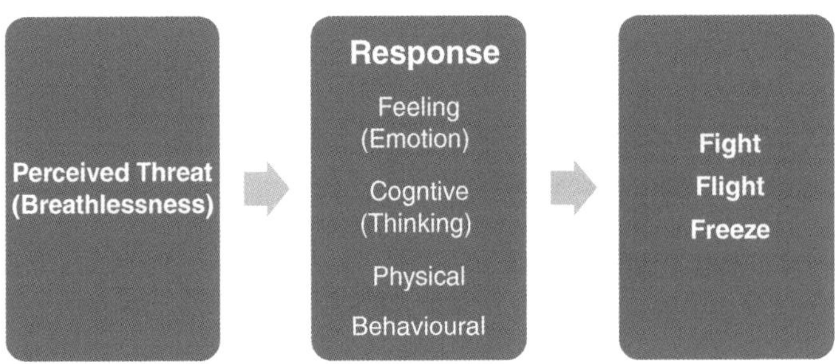

FIGURE 6.1 Fight, flight or freeze response

happens and how strategies can be utilized to control these responses can also make it more likely that the patient will try and use the recommended strategies.

Physical Symptoms

Headaches/Dizziness: Caused by the brain sending a biochemical message to the pituitary gland which releases a hormone that triggers the adrenal gland to release adrenaline. Headaches caused by constriction of the blood vessels in the head.

Blurred Vision: Caused by dilation of the pupils.

Palpitations and Chest Pains: Caused by breathing becoming faster and shallower, supplying more oxygen to the muscles.

Nausea/Indigestion: Caused by digestion being slowed down or stopped by the body as blood is diverted away from the stomach.

Dry Mouth and Difficulty Swallowing: Caused by body fluid such as saliva being redirected into the blood stream.

Aching Muscles: Caused by the large muscles of the body tensing themselves ready for action.

Aching Neck/Back Ache: Caused by the tensing of the muscles in the neck, shoulders and back.

Excess Sweating/Blushing: Caused by the body cooling itself by perspiring. Blood vessels and capillaries move close to the skin's surface.
Rapid Breathing: Caused by the body attempting to supply more and more oxygen to the muscles.
Tingly Skin: Caused by excess oxygen being supplied to the muscles as well as calcium being released from the tense muscles.
Frequent Urination/Diarrhoea: Caused by relaxation of the muscles at the opening of the bladder and sphincter.

The tensing of the muscles of the chest and upper body, increasing heart rate and increased breathing rate are of particular relevance for the breathless patient as these symptoms of anxiety will exacerbate the overall feeling of breathlessness.

Feelings of anxiety can often overwhelm an individual to the extent that they become anxious at the slightest trigger, or anticipation of the trigger, resulting in a disabling fear that can prevent engagement in activity. It is important to spend some time listening noting down the contributing factors to the anxiety, if the person can identify them, and separating them out to facilitate dealing with them one at a time. Addressing issues in this way can help things seem more manageable and this approach is akin to the realistic goal setting outlined in the energy conservation chapter.

How do you eat an elephant? A chunk at a time
African Proverb

Case Study 1
Mr Red is a 64 year old man with Chronic Obstructive Pulmonary Disease. He is experiencing worsening breathlessness and becoming increasing anxious about this, which is having a significant impact on his ability to

function day to day. Mr Red has had recent cardiac investigations which have found no problems with his heart. His recent respiratory review reports stable disease. On assessment Mr Red happened to mention that his father had heart failure and died of a heart attack, "gasping for breath". This is something that Mr Red is terrified of happening to him.

Case Study 2

Mrs Orange is a 57 year old lady with lung cancer. She has recently completed her treatment, and her scan result has indicated a good response. She is now on 3 monthly review with the oncologist. Mrs Orange describes feeling breathless whenever she gets up to do anything. She is extremely frightened about moving as she described how she used to "overdo" it in the garden and read somewhere that this contributed towards her lung cancer diagnosis. She also describes feelings of panic when she is anxious and has asked her GP for oxygen as she had this in hospital and feels this would be useful. Her GP has informed her that she does not need oxygen.

Identifying the Triggers for Anxiety

As a first step it may be helpful to draw up a "vicious daisy" (a technique commonly used in CBT) with the patient whereby all their thoughts, feelings and actions in response to a situation are noted down, an example of which is given in Fig. 6.2. Enabling the patient to take each point in turn presents a more manageable way of addressing each issue in turn and reduces the sense of being overwhelmed by a mass of problems. Being aware of one's limitations as a healthcare professional is imperative when assessing patient's level of and triggers for anxiety and consideration for onward referral to a more appropriate clinician such as a clinical psychologist may be required.

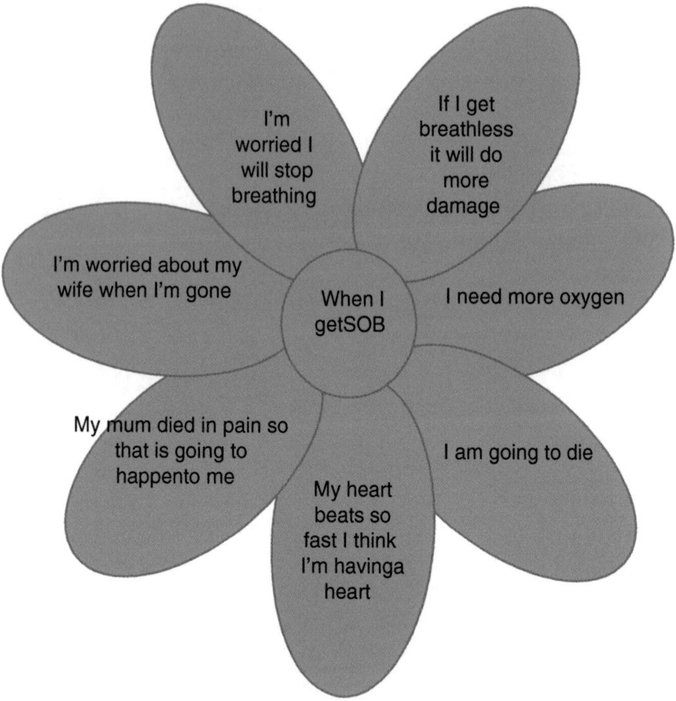

FIGURE 6.2 Vicious daisy

Cognitive Behavioural Therapy

Cognitive Behavioural Therapy (CBT) is an approach which tries to address unhelpful and dysfunctional emotions, thoughts and behaviours. It focuses on what the problems are and the healthcare professional guides discussions to enable the patient to select specific techniques or strategies which help to manage or address these problems. CBT is commonly used to help patients experiencing anxiety or depression and can be an effective approach for helping patients experiencing breathlessness related anxiety. A number of the strategies which can be used for anxiety management with breathlessness patients take some elements of the CBT approach.

However, it may be useful to consider a referral for structured CBT with a qualified professional for patients who have particular and persistent problems with anxiety if they are accepting of this.

Exploring and Dispelling Misperceptions

Many patients with breathlessness will have thoughts which try to provide meaning for why they are breathless and some of these based on fact with others based on experience or their perceptions of a situation. If people have prior experience of a parent or loved one with breathlessness, this can evoke painful and distressing memories each time they become breathless. In the case of Mr Red, his recent cardiac investigation was clear but he still has a very real fear of dying of a heart attack and "gasping for breath", as his father did, although this is unlikely to be the case. Further discussion regarding his fears, and clarifying that his heart investigations were clear, thus making it unlikely that he is going to die of a heart attack when breathless, would perhaps disperse some of these feelings of anxiety and provide reassurance.

It is important to ensure that patients have the correct information and understanding regarding their breathlessness. Explaining and gently challenging their ideas can help to dispel any misperceptions. A common fear that patients have regarding their breathlessness is that they will die "gasping" for breath, when, in reality, this is very unlikely to happen and they are very unlikely to actually stop breathing. Patients find great re-assurance when they were informed that breathlessness, in itself, is not harmful (i.e. it is not harmful to the body to actually be breathless) and that they will recover their breathing. Another common misperception is that breathlessness indicates a need for oxygen whereas the evidence has shown that the use of oxygen does not relieve breathlessness. The use of oxygen saturation monitors can be used to reinforce this point to patients and provide a feedback mechanism to reassure them that their oxygen saturation levels are satisfactory.

Action plan for Breathlessness

I have experienced this before and I am going to recover my breathlessness. I am going to:

Lean forward

Use my fan

Focus on the breath out

I can do it. I am doing it now

FIGURE 6.3 Action plan for breathlessness

Having a Plan of Action

Having identified the triggers for anxiety, it is then useful to work with the patient to try to formulate ways in which to manage these triggers and subsequent sensations in a way that reduces the feelings of anxiety. When feelings of anxiety begin to present themselves, this can result in a inability to think of a clear strategy or plan of management. Sometimes, the use of a simple three point action plan, utilising strategies which can aid recovery of breathlessness, which is kept to hand to be referred to at such times can be very effective (Fig. 6.3). Such action plans can be laminated and placed in areas in which the triggers for anxiety often occur so that they are readily available when required.

Challenging Unhelpful Thoughts

It can be very easy to develop a pattern of thinking unhelpful thoughts or "negative automatic thoughts" which then exacerbate feelings of anxiety and impact greatly on overall well-being. Trying to challenge some of these thoughts can be another effective self-management tool to prevent the exacerbating anxiety. Some of the most common of these thoughts are listed below:

1. "**Always/never**" **thinking** – thinking that bad things "always" happen or that good things "never" happen
2. **Focusing on the negative** – overlooking positive events in favour of focusing on negative ones

3. **Fortune-telling** – predicting that the worst outcome will occur in any given situation
4. **Mind Reading** – the belief one knows what other people are thinking (the interpretation is usually negative)
5. **Constant feelings of guilt** – commonly using words like should, must, ought rather then I would like to or I choose to.
6. **Labelling** – attaching negative labels to oneself, such as "I am so stupid for letting that happen" which can prevent rational thinking about the situation
7. **Personalizing** – attributing negative events or situations to oneself
8. **Blaming** – blaming something or someone else for problems

Relaxation

Relaxation is defined as "the state of being free from tension and anxiety" (Oxford English Dictionary). As individuals, we are unique in the way in which we relax and some understanding of how the breathless patient achieved a state of relaxation prior to feeling breathless is important in informing which relaxation techniques may help them to manage their current level of anxiety. For example, if a person has previously used activities, such as sports or working in the garden, to relieve tension, it may take some time and explanation to enable them to effectively use more sedate forms of relaxation.

Many people may well already employ some strategies to help them to relax, such as reading or listening to a piece of music. Relaxation does not always involve carrying out a structured technique but often using recorded scripts with patients can provide a more organised approached and one which the patient is more likely to adhere to. It is also useful for patients who cannot identify anything that helps them to relax or are new to the concept of relaxation. Sometimes, breathing control techniques, as discussed in Chap. 5, can be a useful way of achieving a state of relaxation. However, in some cases, patients may find that actually focussing on their breathing can increase feelings of anxiety and tension and so it may be helpful to try a relaxation technique prior to then working on their breathing control.

When introducing relaxation techniques to patients, it is vital that the professional feels confident in doing so and has confidence that it can be successful. Patients will often seek reassurance from healthcare professionals, especially when trying something that may be new and unusual for them to try and success in using such techniques will be influenced by the way in which they are introduced and undertaken.

There are a variety of structured relaxation techniques that can be used to manage feelings of anxiety with breathless patients. Those involving actual tensing and relaxing of each group of muscles (such as Jacobson's Progressive Muscular Relaxation) can be useful as a starting point for patients who have never tried relaxation before as this can increase awareness of any areas of muscle tension in the body. Such techniques involve an active tensing of the muscle, then holding this tension, followed by releasing the tension. This is repeated, usually starting from the toes and working up through the body, with the intention of leaving the muscles in a state whereby they are more relaxed than at the start. For patients who are experiencing pain or find it difficult tense the muscle groups, they can be guided to focus on each muscle group in the body but rather than actually tensing the muscles, visualise tensing and releasing the muscles.

Visualisation techniques can also be used to help with anxiety management for the breathless patient. These can be guided, whereby the patient is taken through a particular scene or set of images described, or unguided, whereby the patient is given a few prompts, such as "imagine a favourite place in your mind" but is largely left to imagine their scene to help them achieve a state of relaxation.

Autogenic relaxation, devised by Johannes Schultz and Wolfgang Luthe in the 1930s aims to influence the autonomic nervous system by inducing sensations such as warmth or heaviness in the limbs to reduce muscle tension and reduce the symptoms brought about by the fight, flight, freeze response.

As with any intervention, it is important to carry out a thorough initial assessment as some relaxation techniques may have contraindications. For example autogenic relaxation aims to lower the heart rate and may not be appropriate for patients with some heart conditions. Also, visualisation techniques may be contraindicated for patients with psychotic conditions. To encourage patients to practice relaxation techniques, it may be useful to provide them with a recording which can be played at home. This could either be a generic recording, or a copy of a session which you have carried out with the patient, which may be more meaningful and thus result in the patient being more likely to use it.

Mindfulness

Most people have awareness that if they see or think about something enjoyable, such as chocolate, the very anticipation of eating it can bring pleasure. Mindfulness is a concept derived from Buddhist meditation, although it is often practiced independent of religion. It involves adopting an appreciation and awareness of the "present", trying not to be concerned with what has happened in the past or worrying about what is going to happen in the future. Mindfulness may help to reduce anxiety and once established into a patient's everyday routine and habits, can be a very effective way of managing anxiety associated with breathlessness.

Distraction

Aiding a patient experiencing breathlessness to focus on a situation or image which distracts them from their feelings of anxiety and breathlessness can be a very effective technique in reducing these feelings. This is not to say that it is easy to simply take one's attention away from the anxiety in order to completely remove it. Using visual stimuli, such as a picture frame to help with breathing control (encouraging breathing in for the short side of the frame and breathing out for the longer side) or alternative activities, such as a partner reading a newspaper aloud or talking about an enjoyable time they had together, can be simple but effective tools to use as an interim measure for managing anxiety.

Summary

When drawing up a "vicious daisy" with Mr Red, it would, perhaps, be dominated by thoughts of his fears of dying of a heart attack as his father did. A good starting point would be to reassure him of the results of the recent cardiac investigations and explore how he feels after this. It would also be useful to explain that it would be very unlikely for him to die "gasping for breath" and gently challenging this misperceptions. Other techniques such as relaxation may enable Mr Red to achieve a more relaxed state, which in turn will help management of his breathlessness.

Mrs Orange has just recently completed treatment and it is common for people to feel anxious at this time, particularly when it coincides with longer times in between follow up appointments and less contact with health care professionals. Providing and discussing accurate information regarding the benefits of exercise for breathlessness and challenging the incorrect information regarding the cause of her lung cancer would be a useful first step to try and disperse some of the anxiety triggered by these thoughts. It would also be helpful to talk through her thoughts regarding oxygen, and the fact that it is unlikely to relieve breathlessness, but using other strategies, such as the fan, will provide some relief of breathlessness and a likely impact on reducing anxiety. Having an action plan to refer to and using some form of breathing control or relaxation exercise prior to exercise may also be helpful.

Key Points

- It is important to identify the "triggers" for anxiety
- Try to separate these triggers and focus on them one at a time
- Providing information and education can help to dispel misperceptions and fears, thus reduce anxiety
- Interventions such as relaxation, mindfulness and CBT can be useful in helping to manage anxiety related to breathlessness

- Being aware of one's limitations as a healthcare professional and referring on to relevant clinicians when appropriate is vital

References

Banzett RB, Mulnier HE, Murphy K, Rosen SD, Wise RJ, Adams L. Breathlessness in humans activates insular cortex. Neuroreport. 2000; 11(10):2117–20.

Bausewein C, Booth S, Gysels M, Higginson IJ. Non pharmacological interventions for breathlessness in advanced stages of malignant and non-malignant diseases. Cochrane Database Syst Rev. 2008;(2):CD005623.

Booth S, Moffat C, Burkin J, Galbraith S, Bausewein C. Nonpharmacological interventions for breathlessness. Curr Opin Support Palliat Care. 2011; 5(2):77–86.

Gustavsson C, von Koch L. Applied relaxation in the treatment of long-lasting neck pain: a randomized controlled pilot study. J Rehabil Med. 2006;38(2):100–7.

Hunot V, Churchill R, Teixeira V, Silva de Lima M. Psychological therapies for generalised anxiety disorder (review). Cochrane Collaboration. 2010;(4):CD001848.

Kroner-Herwig B. Chronic pain syndromes and their treatment by psychological interventions. Curr Opin Psychiatry. 2009;22(2):200–4.

Paz-Diaz H, de Oca MM, Lopez JM, Celli BR. Pulmonary rehabilitation improves depression, anxiety, dyspnea and health status in patients with COPD. Am J Phys Med Rehabil. 2007;86(1):30–6.

Thompson B. Mindfulness-based stress reduction for people with chronic conditions. Br J Occup Ther. 2009;72(9):405–10.

Yorke J, Fleming SL, Shuldham C. Psychological interventions for adults with asthma. Cochrane Collaboration. 2009;(1):CD002982.

Chapter 7
Energy Conservation

Evidence
There are few research studies to demonstrate the benefits of energy conservation specifically as a stand-alone intervention (Payne et al. 2012). It is often defined and researched as part of a multidimensional intervention programme, such as pulmonary rehabilitation, for which there is a large body of evidence to support effectiveness (Paz-Diaz et al. 2007). Cognitive Behavioural Therapy also has some evidence to support its effectiveness in the management of breathlessness and reduction in emergency re-admissions for breathlessness patients (Howard et al. 2010). Much of the research refers to energy conservation or activity pacing within the context of Chronic Fatigue Syndrome or pain management (McCracken and Samuel 2007) but this can be equally applied to the breathless patient, regardless of the cause. Booth et al. (2011) acknowledged that whilst energy conservation is frequently used in the management of breathlessness, definition and further research is required. However, energy conservation is an established component of most self-management programmes for breathlessness within the context of long term disease and evidence suggests that such programmes improve confidence to manage breathlessness and reduce hospital admissions (Effing et al. 2009)

S. Booth et al., *Managing Breathlessness in Clinical Practice*, DOI 10.1007/978-1-4471-4754-1_7,

Introduction

Energy conservation and activity pacing are terms that are frequently used interchangeably. How often have we advised a patient to "pace" themselves? Indeed, in the fast pace of life many healthy individuals in the population may have actually received these words of advice. But what does it actually *mean* to pace one's activities? Energy conservation and activity pacing are complex processes of behaviour modification and advising people to do as such, requires changing well established habits and routines; an adjustment which can be difficult and frustrating to achieve. There may also be reluctance in patients and carers to change behaviour if this is interpreted as somehow conceding to the disease process of their long term condition or acknowledgement of the inevitable deterioration.

Breathless patients living with chronic disease often experience fatigue or reduced energy levels which can occur as a consequence of a number of factors. An increase in the severity of pulmonary impairment can lead to a reduction in exercise tolerance, in turn leading to reduced engagement in activities and exercise. This ultimately results in the patient becoming deconditioned to such an extent that activities require more effort and energy to initiate, thus having a major impact on energy levels. In this state, the body is functioning quite inefficiently as the amount of energy expended to carry out day to day tasks is far beyond that used in usual circumstances. Other factors which can come into play are poor appetite (with less "fuel" in the body there is a reduction in energy) and a perceived decline in quality of life which may have a negative influence on mood and, therefore, motivation.

There is often a perceived discourse between energy conservation and exercise, with patients often asking "on the one hand they are telling me to exercise but on the other I am being told to rest, which is right?" Understandably, this can cause confusion and healthcare professionals need to be confident and assured in what the benefits of energy conservation are in order to convincingly advise patients to do it. Energy conservation aims to encourage the most efficient use of energy, which is also one aim of engaging in exercise, therefore the two go hand in hand in managing breathlessness effectively. Whether energy conservation is best achieved by activity pacing, trying to engage more in activity or exercise, adapting activities or a combination of all of these, depends on the lifestyle of the patient.

Facilitating meaningful and useful discussions about energy conservation and encouraging the benefits of such an approach requires an understanding and appreciation of how the person has previously managed their lifestyle and how they are adapting to the change, as well as knowledge of energy conservation techniques.

Case Study

Mr Blue is a 59 year old man with Chronic Obstructive Pulmonary Disease (COPD) He is married and has two adult children who live nearby and visit often. Mr Blue has always worked full-time in a local supermarket and has also led a very active life, cycling to work every day and playing football with his children and grandchildren. He has been on sick leave for the past 6 months due to recurrent exacerbations and increasing breathlessness and is currently consulting with his occupational health department regarding a return to work. Mr Blue wants to return full-time working but his wife feels he should give up work as it is "too much" for him. Mr Blue is expressing frustration at his increasing breathlessness and the limitations it is placing upon his daily activities. He describes himself as a "doer" and has always "been on the go". He is finding it immensely difficult to manage his breathlessness. Yesterday, Mr Blue cleaned all the windows of the house, inside and out, as this is a task that he usually carries out. Today he is exhausted, frustrated and feeling low. Mr and Mrs Blue are finding it increasingly difficult to agree on the way forward, with Mrs Blue thinking that he should rest and "put his feet up" and Mr Blue trying desperately not to "give in to the breathlessness".

All or Nothing

One central principle to encourage is obtaining balance between activity and rest. Identifying where a patient is on this continuum is helpful. A clinical observation of some patients is that they often fall into a pattern of excessive activity when they have a good day, only to have this followed by a few days of feeling exhausted and not being able to do anything. It is natural to want to make the most of feeling well and often patients are at their most resourceful on these days. However, their immediate gratification of having pushed themselves to the limit can be followed by subsequent days of feeling frustrated and low at having no energy. This pattern of behaviour can be described as the "all or nothing" or "boom or bust" approach and patients or carers will often immediately relate to this when it is highlighted.

Whilst, on occasion, this is difficult to avoid, for example if there is a family event such as a wedding or if the patient has several unavoidable appointments all in one go, it is a pattern that is helpful to discourage. Using energy in this way can be very inefficient. If patients push themselves to the limit, they are running the risk of becoming run down and possibly picking up infections which, in the case of COPD, can be very detrimental. It can often take longer to recover from these periods of over exertion which can result in an accumulative reduction in activity participation over time due to the time required to recover.

Explaining that it is far better to do a little less on the good days in order to be able to do a little more on the not so good days is a worthy piece of advice that many patients, once they have agreed to adjust their pattern of activity, find extremely useful. Using an analogy of an elastic band can also be helpful, suggesting that if you stretch the band too far, it is at risk of becoming frayed and eventually snapping.

Activity Participation Habits

For those patients who are used to living a very sedentary life, energy conservation still involves balancing activity and rest and also requires an adjustment in lifestyle but it is more about trying to encourage engagement in some form of activity rather than advising restraint. Encouraging this modification in behaviour can be as much of a challenge as advising someone who has an "all or nothing" approach. It is imperative to start at the point of explaining that one of the keys to managing a reduction in energy levels, and in turn managing breathlessness, is to try and use the body in the most efficient way possible. Engaging in an activity or exercise, as explained in more detail in Chap. 8, enables the muscles to be used more efficiently and, therefore, utilises energy in a better way.

> Energy Conservation aims to use the body in the most efficient way possible. They are complimentary techniques in the management of breathlessness.

Establishing what kind of activities the patient enjoys or previously enjoyed is important as trying to encourage them to engage in a pleasurable or meaningful activity will be more motivating than simply asking them to "do more" when they have no inclination or drive to do so. A further helpful strategy can be to incorporate an activity into the usual routine, such as a walk in the garden if they are putting the rubbish out, or if going out in a wheelchair with relatives, spending some of the time walking with the wheelchair rather than sitting in it for the duration of the outing.

Adapting Activities

In order to understand energy conservation and activity pacing, it is important to appreciate the concept of activity, as any effective intervention regarding pacing involves the analysis of activity (breaking down its component parts) and trying to simplify components where possible to conserve energy. As clinicians expressly skilled in the analysis of activity, occupational therapists focus on the pattern of activities, the meaning and purpose that people place on them and the impact that illness has on the ability to carry them out so it is worth considering a referral to an occupational therapist if this is possible.

In self-management of breathlessness, the goal is for the patient to be able to develop strategies to enable coping with an often changing situation. By breaking down activities and simplifying where possible, this can help the patient to remain independent by continuing to carry out the activity but in a different way. Many people describe mornings as being their worst time of day and making a few minor changes such as sitting down to wash, looking at positioning in the shower to incorporate a forward lean position, using a handheld fan positioned on the basin or opening a window whilst brushing teeth, can be helpful techniques to manage breathlessness at this time. When providing meals, it may be that the patient has the energy to prepare the food but not to cook it, so agreeing a plan with the family can be a useful strategy.

Appropriate use of equipment can assist with activity pacing and serve to conserve energy which can then be used at a later stage. For example, bath aids to enable patients to get in and out of the bath more easily can help conserve energy for both the patient and carer to the degree that they have more energy to engage in other activities such as going out with family or going for a walk later in the day. Discussions regarding equipment provision need sensitive handling to aid acceptance and patient confidence.

Activity Pacing

We have already discussed the difficulties of modifying behaviour and doing things in a different way. However, pacing oneself can often lead to a more satisfying lifestyle which can encourage a sense of achievement rather than a sense of continued pressure and failure to succeed.

> Actions such as slowing the rate of walking, taking time to enjoy one's surroundings, or cleverly using park benches or seats within a shopping centre can all be used to help pace one's walking.

Also useful is preparing others, so if an event or appointment is coming up, allowing extra time to get ready or informing others that it is going to take a bit longer in the morning can be helpful. It is far better to advise patients to take longer to do something and complete it rather than being too exhausted to finish it.

Prioritising

It is important to gauge which activities are a priority for the patient as these will be the ones which they are eager to maintain, and therefore the ones which require attention. Sometimes it is useful to ask patients to list down their activities and then prioritise them in order of low, medium and high priority. This may in the first instance demonstrate how many things they are trying to take on, if they have a very long list, but also focuses them on thinking about how they want to use their energy.

Analogies are often a good way of explaining how to use and conserve energy and to identify priorities, as in the earlier example of the elastic band. Ask patients to think about a simple envelope. Prior to experiencing breathlessness they may have had an A4 sized envelope; if they put all the activities that they need or wish to do on pieces of paper, these would all fit nicely in the envelope. Now that they are experiencing breathlessness, they have a smaller envelope (A5) and it is not possible to fit in all of the pieces of paper (i.e. all of their activities) so which ones are priorities and which ones do they need to delegate, do differently or discard? Another way of helping to prioritise energy is to ask the patient to imagine having a jug of energy for each day. This jug is topped up overnight. What do they want to use this jug of energy on? Once the jug is empty, there is no energy left. There are things that may top the energy jug up, such as relaxation or restorative activities such as painting or craft work but most activities will expend the energy and this is a useful way of encouraging patients to think about their energy levels and using their energy in a more efficient way.

Realistic Goal Setting

Encouraging patients to set realistic and achievable goals can enable them to manage and use their energy in a more efficient way as well as facilitating a sense of achievement. Once a patient's priorities have been established, goal setting can be an efficient way of focusing on those things which provide meaning and purpose for the patient. The role of the healthcare professional in this process is to ensure that the patient has set a goal that will enable them to achieve the required outcome, and facilitating discussion around making the goal more realistic if they have chosen something that it beyond their capabilities.

Planning

Although it appears obvious, planning activities around the best times for the patient is vital not only to utilising energy in the most efficient way but also enabling maximal enjoyment of these activities. Where possible it is helpful to advise planning activities in advance, for example if the patient is going out to meet with friends in a restaurant, does the restaurant have stairs, are the toilets easily accessible, is there a more private area to sit which may be preferred if the patient is particularly conscious of their breathlessness.

Not everyone is keen or motivated to plan activities in advance but it can be a very useful way of preventing unnecessary energy being exerted and once integrated into a daily routine can become an established pattern of behaviour.

Posture

A surprising amount of excess energy can be expended through adopting poor postures. Positions to ease breathlessness are discussed in more detail in Chap. 4, but it is worth considering assessing patients when carrying out various tasks or activities to establish whether a change in posture or positioning could assist with conserving or more efficient use of energy and helping the patient to relieve their breathlessness. Adopting the positions to ease breathlessness when carrying out functional tasks, such as using the *forward lean* position when pushing a shopping trolley round the supermarket or when going to the toilet can be a useful way of using energy more efficiently as can use of equipment or devices, such as a powered backrest to aid an elevated position when in bed which can relieve breathlessness.

Sleep

Gaining an understanding of a patient's sleep wake cycle and establishing whether there have been any changes in this may provide some useful information with regard to reduced energy levels. If patients are having difficulty sleeping at night and this is a change to the usual routine, it is helpful to see if the patient can identify the reason why this is happening, if there are any immediate solutions to ease the problem, such as liaising with the GP with regard to timing of medications if these are contributing to sleep disturbances or providing a urinal bottle to use rather than having to get up several times to use the toilet. Sleep enhancing medications can also be helpful in these situations where appropriately prescribed.

Sleeping during the day, if this is a change to the usual routine, should be discouraged where possible, or at least kept to a minimum of 20–30 min naps. If a pattern of sleeping during the day is emerging, some patients may be happy to allow a carer or relative or set an alarm to ensure that they have a short nap rather than a prolonged sleep. Other strategies to manage breathlessness, such as engaging in exercise or relaxation may have a beneficial effect on helping the person to sleep. Behaviours such as trying to avoid caffeine immediately before going to bed, trying to have a milky drink, maintaining a comfortable temperature in the bedroom, and using essential oils, such as lavender, may help to relax and consequentially aid sleep. If the patient is having difficulty getting back to sleep and spending many hours lying awake in bed, advise them to get up out of bed, make a drink for themselves, and then try going back to bed to sleep, thus trying to break the association of going to bed with endless hours lying awake.

Effective Rest

Energy conservation involves getting a balance between activity and rest and it is useful to encourage the idea of "effective" rest with activities such as relaxation or craft activities; those which aim to relax the mind and body and rejuvenate. Helping to identify sources of and manage anxiety and stress in order to be able to truly rest is vital and this is discussed further in chapter 6. Effective use of energy conservation techniques will hopefully have an impact on the patient's overall well-being with the aim being to enable them to have the control and ability to engage in pleasurable activities. Encouraging patients to spend time outside, if possible, can have a positive impact on their general health and sense of well-being. It is also worth acknowledging to patients that it is acceptable to do things in a different way, or not at all, which may be difficult for them to accept if they are habits and routines which have been established over a lifetime.

Summary

So, let us come back to Mr Blue. Here we clearly have someone who has adopted an "all or nothing" approach to life with the added complexity of his wife wanting him to rest more as she thinks he is doing too much. It would be important to explain the concept of balancing activity and rest and encouraging the idea of doing a little less on the good days in order to be able to do more on the not so good days, and in turn be able to do more over time. Using the analogies of the elastic band and the energy jar may help in trying to explain the reason why he is feeling exhausted today. It might also be useful to discuss the work situation and encourage a more graded return to work rather than an immediate return to full time working. Mr Blue clearly enjoys exercise and activity and so a graded exercise programme is likely to be something that he would engage in. Talking through adjusting to a changing situation is going to be key in agreeing an achievable goal for Mr Blue and will also need the support and backing of Mrs Blue.

Key Points

1. Energy conservation requires a change in behaviour and this can be difficult to accept and achieve
2. Understanding how a person has previously managed their lifestyle is **fundamental** to knowing what advice will be most helpful
3. Energy conservation involves getting a balance between activity and rest
4. Energy conservation aims to utilise energy in the most efficient way possible
5. Energy conservation is an important component in effective self-management of breathlessness

References

Booth S, Moffat C, Burkin J, Galbraith S, Bausewein C. Nonpharmacological interventions for breathlessness. Curr Opin Support Palliat Care. 2011;5(2):77–86.

Effing T, Monninkhof EEM, van der Valk PP, Zielhuis GGA, Walters EH, van der Palen JJ, Zwerink M. Self-management education for patients with chronic obstructive pulmonary disease (Review). The Cochrane Collaboration. Issue 4; 2009:CD002990.

Howard C, Dupont S, Haselden B, Lynch J, Wills P. The effectiveness of a group cognitive-behavioural breathlessness intervention on health status, mood and hospital admission in elderly patients with chronic obstructive pulmonary disease. Psychol Health Med. 2010;15(4): 371–85.

McCracken LM, Samuel VM. The role of avoidance, pacing and other activity patterns in chronic pain. Pain. 2007;130(1–2):119–25.

Payne C, Wiffen PJ, Martin S. Interventions for fatigue and weight loss in adults with advanced progressive illness (Review). The Cochrane Collaboration. Issue 8; 2012:CD008427.

Paz-Diaz H, de Oca MM, Lopez JM, Celli BR. Pulmonary rehabilitation improves depression, anxiety, dyspnea and health status in patients with COPD. Am J Phys Med Rehabil. 2007;86(1):30–6.

Part IV
Non-pharmacological Interventions – Functioning

Chapter 8
Exercise and Activity Promotion

"When I found out I'd got cancer, you think 'I'm ill', whereas she made me see that you can still do exercise, all the exercises that you can do and when she left I felt much more confident actually, I did definitely"

–A patient with lung cancer

Introduction

Regular exercise and activity has been proven to improve breathlessness however breathless patients often avoid exercise and activity due to the misguided fear that breathlessness is harmful. Some patients may avoid exertion simply just to avoid this unpleasant symptom. Carers may also re-enforce negative beliefs regarding exercise, therefore promoting a sedentary life style. Inactivity may cause the breathless patient to become deconditioned and their breathlessness may worsen as a result. The clinician's role is to address barriers to exercise and promote regular, appropriate exercise and activity. This chapter will introduce and explore a step-wise process to exercise and activity promotion to help guide the clinician to empower the breathless patient to engage in lifelong exercise and activity.

S. Booth et al., *Managing Breathlessness in Clinical Practice*,
DOI 10.1007/978-1-4471-4754-1_8,

Evidence and Guidelines Regarding Exercise in Breathlessness Management

Pulmonary rehabilitation has been proven to reduce breathlessness (National Clinical Guideline Centre 2010). Exercise may reduce breathlessness by improving cardiopulmonary efficiency. Exercise, during a pulmonary rehabilitation programme, may also 'desensitise' the flight-fight response of primitive brain centres to the sensation of breathlessness, through the combination of repeated, self-induced exertional breathlessness in a safe environment, alongside breathlessness management education, enabling the patient to effectively self manage this normally distressing symptom. In overweight patients exercise, alongside dietary advice, may also help to improve breathlessness by reducing excess weight and therefore reduce the physical demands on the cardiovascular system.

Exercise is widely promoted in national guidelines for a variety of long-term conditions in which breathlessness is a symptom, based on the strength of evidence supporting its use. Disease specific group-based exercise rehabilitation programmes have been recommended in the guidelines for chronic obstructive pulmonary disease (COPD) (National Clinical Guideline Centre 2010), idiopathic pulmonary fibrosis (National Institute for Health and Clinical Excellence (NICE) 2013) and chronic heart failure (NICE 2010).

Cardiac rehabilitation is often more intense than pulmonary rehabilitation, therefore pulmonary rehabilitation may be more suitable for patients with chronic heart failure. Evans et al. (2007) demonstrated that it is feasible for patients with chronic heart failure to attend pulmonary rehabilitation alongside COPD patients and to make comparable improvements to the patients with COPD. Physical training, to improve cardiopulmonary efficiency, is also promoted in the management of asthma (British Thoracic Society /Scottish Intercollegiate Guidelines Network (BTS/SIGN) 2012).

Exercise training for patients post cancer treatment provides both physiological and psychological beneficial effect (Spence et al. 2010; Speck et al. 2010). Pulmonary rehabilitation has been shown to improve exercise tolerance and functional status in oncology patients with pulmonary symptoms (Morris et al. 2009). Exercise training is considered to be safe during and after cancer treatment and results in improvements in quality of life, physical functioning and cancer related fatigue and inactivity should be avoided even in those with current disease or undergoing difficult treatment (American College of Sports Medicine (ACSM) 2010).

The Clinician's Role in Exercise and Activity Promotion

Guidelines generally advocate exercise alongside education in a group setting, in preference to individual home exercise programmes. Group work provides peer support which may improve motivation, as well as providing the opportunity for regular supervised exercise in a safe and supportive environment. Puente-Maestu et al. (2000) showed that a supervised exercise training programme produce significantly greater physiological improvements in exercise tolerance than a self motivated programme for patients with COPD.

Proven Benefits of Pulmonary Rehabilitation Programmes for COPD

- Improved exercise tolerance
- Reduced breathlessness
- Improved quality of life
- Improvements in healthcare utilisation
- Improvements in psychological outcomes

BTS/ACPRC (2009)

Ultimately the clinician should strive to engage the breathless patient in an exercise-based rehabilitation programme specific to their condition. However not all patients feel ready to attend a group programme due to lack of confidence, severely reduced exercise tolerance or fear of uncontrolled breathlessness. The clinician's role may therefore be to assist the patient to make the transition to an appropriate group exercise programme.

Conversely some patients may not wish to attend a group out of personal choice or there may not be a suitable and accessible programme available to the patient, the patient may be 'too fit' or not 'fit enough'. Other patients may have attended a group programme but have not continued an exercise regime, in such cases patients may be able to repeat the programme if local commissioning allows and the patient wishes. In cases where a rehabilitation programme is not suitable, available or is declined alternative exercise strategies need to be explored and put in place.

A Stepwise Approach to Exercise and Activity Promotion

It can be difficult to know where to begin with the daunting task of exercise and activity promotion in the breathless patient. A stepwise process is therefore suggested to help guide the clinician (Fig. 8.1).

Steps to exercise and activity promotion

- **Step 1:** Explain the deconditioning cycle to the patient and their carer and the fact deconditioning can be 'reversed' through exercise and increased activity.
- **Step 2:** Explore the patient's individual fears and barriers to exercise.
- **Step 3:** Explore the patient's motivation for exercise and set goals.
- **Step 4:** Provide advice and education on techniques to manage breathlessness on exertion.
- **Step 5:** Engage the patient in a suitable exercise programme or personal regime.
- **Step 6:** Ensure ongoing monitoring of progress, support regarding goals and continued motivation

FIGURE 8.1 Steps to exercise and activity promotion

Step 1: Deconditioning Cycle

Patients who are breathless due to pathology may fear that breathlessness is harmful and therefore avoid becoming breathless. This leads to inactivity and the downward spiral of deconditioning (Celli 2009).

> Patients and their carers need to be reassured that breathlessness in itself is not harmful. Indeed, making themselves moderately breathless with activity is actually improving their cardiovascular health.

> Patients need to understand that the more 'unfit' they are the more breathless they will feel on activity.

Before embarking on exercise and activity promotion it is important to ensure the patient understands this deconditioning cycle (Fig. 8.2). It is also important to help patients

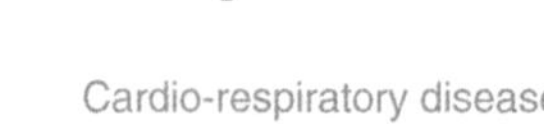

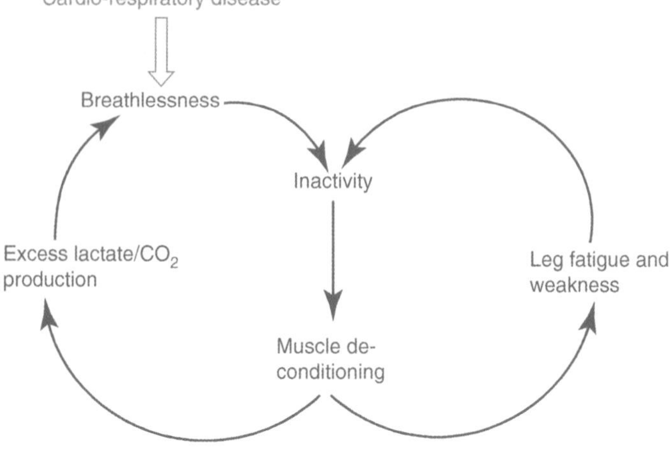

FIGURE 8.2 Deconditioning cycle

and carers recognise the effect of specific periods of reduced activity, which may be related to being unwell with an exacerbation, hospital admission or the winter months when they may be less active outside and how breathlessness may be noticeably worse following such periods due to reduced cardiopulmonary fitness and general loss of strength.

> Chronic conditions cannot be reversed or cured, however cardiopulmonary endurance, general strength and flexibility are all things that patients can have a positive influence upon.

It can be very empowering for patients to realise that improving fitness is one of the things they can influence to make a positive difference to their lives, at a time when they may feel at the mercy of their condition.

Exercise and activity promotion is a vital part of breathlessness self management. By reversing the 'deconditioning cycle' through improving cardiovascular endurance, muscle strength and endurance and general flexibility patients may find they may become less breathless on exertion and recover quicker. Regular exercise may also improve mood though release of endorphins.

Exercise causing 'deliberate' breathlessness can provide an opportunity for patients to practice their breathlessness management techniques in a safe support environment where they feel in control. Regular exercise where breathlessness is self induced but the patient feels in control and not anxious may help to 'desensitise' the fight-flight response of the primitive brain centres to the perception of breathlessness.

Step 2: Overcoming Common Barriers to Exercise

Often the biggest barrier to exercise is motivation, confidence and self-belief in the ability to carry out regular, meaningful exercise that will have a positive influence to symptoms and daily life. Patients may also have specific barriers to exercise, which they may discuss openly or disguise behind vague excuses. It is important to discover the real reasons for exercise avoidance so that these barriers can be explored and addressed (see Table 8.1).

Barriers Created by Carers

Some barriers maybe created or re-enforced by the patient's carer therefore discussion regarding exercise should include the patient's carer.

> Well meaning carers may find it distressing to see their loved one 'fighting for breath' and may encourage the patient to rest and thereby re-enforcing the sedentary life-style.

TABLE 8.1 Common barriers to exercise

Barrier	Possible solutions
Fear that breathlessness or exercise is harmful.	Explain the deconditioning cycle, that breathlessness is not harmful and it is normal to become breathless when exercising. In fact it is important to become breathless with exercise to improve fitness. Demonstrate oxygen levels stay within normal range or recover within acceptable time (with oxygen if prescribed long term or ambulatory), therefore it is the effort of breathing, not low oxygen that causes breathlessness.
Motivation, especially in the context of frequent exacerbations.	Explain to the patient that research shows that even if pulmonary rehabilitation is interrupted by an exacerbation of COPD they can still achieved similar outcomes to those who completed the course without interruption (Steel et al. 2010). Explain deconditioning cycle and the fact it can be reversed through exercise. Use goal setting, starting with simple, achievable goals.
Lack of confidence to exercise.	Discuss specific cause of reduced confidence. What do they fear will happen? Start with small achievable goals using exercise patient feels most confident with. Exercise with a friend. Attend supervised exercise group specific to their condition or a seated exercise group. May wish just to observe group first.
Fear of infection, often related to group work, gym or swimming pool.	Exercise outdoors or at home with own equipment. Take disinfection wipes and clean equipment before use. Some patients may feel more comfortable in a small, private swimming pool i.e. at health club or hotel.
Fear of not being able to keep up with rest of class.	Observe class before attending. One to one assessment with instructor prior to course so can try out exercise circuit. Build up exercise tolerance prior to starting class with home exercise or walking programme. Attend basic seated exercise class first and build up from there.

Table 8.1 (continued)

Barrier	Possible solutions
Fear breathlessness will become uncontrolled during exercise.	Gain confidence in breathlessness self management strategies, such as breathing techniques, with low intensity exercise at first and build up gradually as confidence improves. Ensure the patient understands breathlessness will recover with rest. Discuss previous situations where patient felt breathlessness was uncontrolled. What would they do differently next time?
Weather; too cold, hot, windy etc.	On such days exercise indoors i.e. home exercise programme, interactive games console, DVD, exercise class at a sports centre, swimming, gym, walking around shopping centres or supermarkets.
Logistics of getting to venue.	Go with a friend or relative. Access volunteer driver scheme. Reduced price taxis for those with disabilities/ chronic conditions. NHS transport. Ask organiser if there is anyone who lives near them who could car share or what transport arrangements are available. Home exercise, interactive games console, DVD, walking programme.
Pain, fatigue, weakness.	Pain should be addressed. Joint pain and stiffness from arthritis may be helped by appropriate exercise. Fatigue and weakness should also improve with exercise. Although patients may initially feel more fatigued when starting exercise until their fitness improves.
Unsure what exercise to do, especially if very low exercise tolerance.	Simple bed, chair or standing exercise at home. Build up exercise in 10 min sessions. Getting up and walking the length of the room or corridor every 1–2 h, maybe combined with a pedometer. Seated exercise class. Bowls or other low level sport. Interval training (exercise interspersed with short periods of rest or lower intensity exercise). Neuromuscular electrical stimulation. Inspiratory muscle training.

(continued)

TABLE 8.1 (continued)

Barrier	Possible solutions
Cost of exercise instruction or equipment.	Subsidised schemes such as GP gym exercise referral, personal health coach or exercise for over 50 years old or those with chronic conditions. Walking programme with or without low cost pedometer. Home exercise programme with or without DVD. Exercise programmes run by charities or the National Health Service.
Previous bad experience when exercising or blames exercise for deterioration in their condition.	Discuss and rationalise what happened and why. Discuss how such a situation could be managed in the future. Try a different sort of exercise or activity unrelated to past event. Cognitive behavioural therapy.

If possible the carer should observe the patient exercising and recovering their breathing after exercising to help reduce the carer's fear and anxiety related to their loved one exercising. In appropriate cases both carer and patient attending an exercise class or exercising together (i.e. taking regular walks) may aid motivation and the patient's confidence to exercise as well as benefiting the carer themselves.

Step 3: Goal Setting

Goals aid motivation by giving a sense of purpose and the 'feel good' factor of achievement. Goals must be set based on the patient's motivation, not what the clinician or carer thinks is best for the patient. Set just one or two goals at a time to aid focus. Goals must be SMART: Specific, Measurable, Achievable, Realistic and Timed. For example "To become fitter" is not a SMART goal. Sort terms goals may lead to an overall long term goal.

Long Term Goal

To be able to walk to the corner shop (50 m away) three times a week by 1 month time.

Short Term Goals

Week 1: To walk three times a week 20 m (to the lamp post) and back.
Week 2: To walk three times a week 30 m (to the bin) and back.
Week 3: To walk three times a week 40 m (to the park gate) and back.

Goals should be written in a positive manner. For example "I will iron for 10 min each day" not "I will not fall behind with the ironing". To help goals to be realistic ask patients to rate how confident they feel, out of ten, that they will achieve the goal. If their confidence level is less than seven then the patient should re-think the goal. It can help to monitor progress in a diary so patients can see that they are making progress towards their goal. Patients should reward themselves for achieving their goal. This does not have to be a grand or expensive celebration. Going out for lunch with their partner or coffee with a friend, going to the cinema or theatre, buying a new item of clothing or treating themselves to a massage, new book or DVD. The patient then needs to set their next goal.

Explaining how exercise can help a patient achieve their goals and enable them to see the relevance of exercise in their life aids motivation. Exercise diaries and goal setting sheets are produced by charities such as Macmillan Cancer Support, the British Lung Foundation and the British Heart Foundation.

Step 4: Managing Breathlessness on Exertion

A common fear of both patient and carer is that breathlessness may become uncontrolled during exercise and that this may lead the patient to become 'stranded' if on a walk, embarrassed if in an exercise class or in a public place or they may fear breathlessness will cause them harm. Prior to commencing on a programme of exercise it is important that patients are confident in using breathlessness self management techniques to manage exertional breathlessness and that their carer can observe that such techniques are successful.

Managing Exertional Breathlessness

- **Education**: Understand breathlessness is not harmful. In fact becoming moderately breathless during exercise will help improve cardiopulmonary fitness. Breathlessness will recover with rest.
- **Cool draught of air**: Fan to the face, cool mist spray or flannel to wet face during and post exercise.
- **Breathing techniques**: Paced breathing in time with steps or movement, breathe out on effort, Breathing Control, Recovery Breathing, pursed-lips breathing. Practice techniques at rest initially to become familiar and competent, then use during activity to manage breathlessness. Gradually increase intensity of breathlessness as confidence in technique improves.
- **Positions**: Adjust position during exercise to avoid supine positions, bending at waist or abdominal compression. Positions during exercise or post exercise that help utilise breathing accessory muscles, such as the forward lean position and upper limb bracing.
- **Walking aid**: Use of walking stick as a portable leaning post or walking frame to maintain the forward lean position while on the move.
- **Pharmacology**: Trial of bronchodilator (if prescribed as required) 20–30 min prior to exercise to see if reduces exertional breathlessness. Use oxygen during

exercise if prescribed for long term or ambulatory use. Patients prescribed short burst oxygen therapy may find using oxygen during exercise may prolong the duration they are able to exercise. A trial of exercise with and without oxygen may clarify this. Discuss with the patient's oxygen prescriber if a change of oxygen prescription is indicated.
- **Warm up and cool down**: May help patient to adjust and manage breathlessness sensation.
- **Build up gradually**: Start with easily achievable exercise and then increase over weeks as confidence grows.
- **Progress**: Ensure patients are still achieving moderate breathlessness during exercise to ensure optimal benefit as they progress.

Step 5: Engage the Patient in a Suitable Exercise Programme or Regime

I think the most important thing of all was the exercises. I make a point of doing them every morning for 10 min if I can. If I find that after 10 min I'm a bit puffy I sit down for quarter of an hour and then I'll have another try. Now I can do 10 min without sitting down, so I have improved. – A gentleman with pulmonary fibrosis.

Prior to commencing any new exercise routine the patient should be screened for contraindications and precautions to the proposed exercise or activity, warned of possible adverse effects and what to do if these occur. They should also have any prescribed medication, such as glyceryl trinitrate (GTN) spray or bronchodilator inhalers, nearby when exercising.

The Department of Health has made recommendations regarding the amount of exercise and activity adults should achieve each week. These recommendations may also act as an aspiration to people with long-term conditions. It has been recommended that cancer survivors should be advised to gradually build up to these physical activity guidelines (Campbell et al. 2012). For those with very advanced chronic disease this may not be a realistic target, however this group may still be able to accumulate 30 min of appropriate physical activity in three bouts of 10 min a day. The intensity and type of activity should be appropriate to the patient and patients with very low levels of exercise tolerance would need to build up to this level of activity.

Department of Health Exercise & Activity Recommendation for Adults (2011)

- 150 min of moderate activity over a week.
- Suggests 150 min maybe split into 30 min, 5 days a week.
- Can accumulate in sets of 10 min or more a day.
- Undertake muscle strength training on at least 2 days a week.
- Minimise the time spent sedentary (sitting).

Older adults (65 years or older) who are at risk of falls should include balance and co-ordination exercise on at least 2 days a week.

Considerations When Choosing an Exercise or Activity

Appropriate: Does the exercise or activity address the patient's needs and goals? i.e. a yoga class does not improve cardiovascular fitness.

Suitable: Are there any precautions or contraindications? Is the intensity of exercise or activity at the right level for the patient?

Feasible: Affordable? accessible?

Sustainable: Does the patient have the time, motivation and means to continue the exercise or activity long term?
Enjoyable: The most important consideration if the exercise or activity is to be continued long term. Take a friend!

Examples of Types of Exercise
Cardiovascular: Walking, jogging, running, bike, rower, aerobics class or DVD, dancing, swimming.
Strength training: Free weights, weight machines.
Balance, co-ordination, flexibility: Tai Chi, yoga, dancing.
Impact (consider to maintain bone strength): Walking, step ups, jogging, running, dancing, aerobics class.

Pulmonary Rehabilitation Guidelines for COPD
(American Thoracic Society & European Respiratory Society (ATS & ERS) 2006)

- Minimum 20 sessions in total. 3 sessions a week, 1 session a week can be unsupervised.
- Cardiovascular exercise; work at greater than 60 % of maximum work rate, (correlates with 4–6 on modified Borg scale for breathlessness) for at least 30 min, if possible. This high intensity exercise provides greatest benefit and should be encouraged, however low intensity exercise still has a training effect in those who cannot manage high intensity.
- Interval training (longer exercise sessions broken down into several shorter sessions with rest or low intensity exercise in between) maintains training effect but with less symptoms and therefore may promote a higher level of exercise training in more symptomatic patents.
- Strength training is worthwhile.

Strength Training

- Strength training should consist of 2–4 sets of 6–12 repetitions at an intensity of 50–85 % of 1 repetition max (1RM) (i.e. percentage of the maximal weight the person can lift once through full range) (O'Shea et al. 2004). For untrained elderly start at 50 % intensity.
- Strength training should occur on 2–3 days a week and include the major muscles of trunk and limbs including pectoralis major, lattissimus dorsi, trapezius, deltoid, biceps, triceps, quadriceps and hamstrings (Benton and Swan 2006).

1 Repetition Max (1 RM) Test Procedure (Benton and Swan 2006)

1. Light warm up of 5–10 repetitions for 40–60 % perceived maximum.
2. 1 min rest, then perform 3–5 repetitions at 60–80 % perceived maximum (should be close to perceived 1 RM).
3. A small amount of weight added and a 1 RM lift attempted.
4. If successful, rest for 3–5 min then repeat with slightly heavier weight.
5. Aim to find 1 RM in 3–5 attempts.
6. 1 RM is the weight of the last successfully reported lift.

Recording Exercise and Activity

It is important to record exercise and activity in order to help guide their routine, motivate the patient and enable them to see progress. The modified Borg scale (Fig. 8.3), originally designed to measure exertion, is commonly used in pulmonary rehabilitation to rate breathlessness during exertion in order to help the patient exercise at the correct intensity to improve their cardiovascular fitness. Patients are usually advised to maintain their perceived breathlessness during exercise at between 4–6 on the Borg scale.

Modified Borg Scale

Score	Severity of breathlessness
0	No breathlessness at all
0.5	Very, very slight (just noticeable)
1	Very slight breathlessness
2	Slight breathlessness
3	Moderate breathlessness
4	Somewhat severe breathlessness
5	Severe breathlessness
6	
7	Very severe breathlessness
8	
9	Almost maximum breathlessness
10	Maximum breathlessness

Borg (1982)

FIGURE 8.3 Modified Borg scale

	Mon	Tues	Wed	Thurs	Fri	Sat	Sun
Sit to stand							
Repetitions							
Borg							
Bicep Curls							
Reps/weight							
Borg							

FIGURE 8.4 Example of part of an exercise diary

Some patients may struggle to rate their breathlessness using the modified Borg scale. In such cases it may help to describe ‘moderate’ intensity exercise as breathless enough that you can still talk but not in full sentences or that you can talk but not sing or that you feel you are breathless and working hard but you don’t need to ‘reach for your inhaler’.

The maximal Borg score is recorded for each exercise in an exercise diary (Fig. 8.4). Patients may notice their Borg score reduce as they become more fit. The clinician should therefore ensure the patient works a little harder to maintain their Borg score at the specified level i.e. work faster, more repetitions or increase weight so they lift a greater percentage 1 repetition max (1RM).

Simple and cheap weights may be created from filling plastic milk bottles with water or stones. These have a convenient handle and the amount of weight placed within the bottle can be easily adjusted as required. It is important to include a warm up and cool down, stretches for muscles used during exercise and general neck, shoulder, thoracic cage and spine mobility exercises as these areas may become stiff in those with breathlessness or chronic lung conditions. A poor posture can restrict lung expansion and exacerbate breathlessness. Particular attention should be paid to improving posture, which may have adapted into a 'chin poke', 'slumped spine' and 'rounded, hunched shoulders' posture due to chronic overuse of breathing accessory muscles. Stretches for tight muscles, shoulder girdle retraction with scapular setting and deep neck flexor strengthening may be required alongside posture advice.

Patients with severe COPD may not be able to exercise to the intensity to induce a cardiovascular training effect however studies suggest that exercise benefit is independent of the degree of impairment, so that even severe COPD patients should benefit from appropriate exercise (Celli 2009).

Patients who are unable or unwilling to attend a pulmonary rehabilitation or group exercise programme may benefit from an appropriate home exercise programme. Exercise programmes based on COPD group pulmonary rehabilitation programmes have been shown to be effective in a variety of long-term conditions such as cancer, pulmonary fibrosis and chronic heart failure (Evans et al. 2007; Morris et al. 2009, NICE 2010, 2013). It is therefore feasible that a home exercise programme based on the pulmonary rehabilitation guidelines given above may provide a 'stepping stone' in order to build confidence and eventually enable the patient to attend pulmonary rehabilitation or other suitable group exercise. DVDs and interactive games consoles may help motivate patients carrying out home exercise.

Inspiratory Muscle Training

Inspiratory muscle strength has been shown to correlate with exercise performance in those with incurable thoracic cancer

(England et al. 2012). Inspiratory muscle training (IMT) in those with COPD has been shown to improve inspiratory muscle strength and endurance, functional exercise capacity, dyspnoea and quality of life (Gosselink et al. 2011). IMT is recommended in the BTS/ACPRC (2009) guidelines for COPD but should not replace pulmonary rehabilitation unless the patient is unable or unwilling to partake in pulmonary rehabilitation. It is possible that self induced increased work of breathing and breathlessness via regular IMT sessions, while the patient remains calm and fully in control, may dampen down the flight-fight response of primitive brain centres to the sensation breathlessness.

Case Study: Home Exercise

Mrs Jones is a 59 year old lady with severe emphysema. She has been out of hospital for 2 months following a 40 day admission to ITU for type II respiratory failure. Ambulatory oxygen therapy prescribed and Mrs Jones also monitors her own oxygen saturations. Mrs Jones was anxious about becoming breathless; "You're not going to make me climb the stairs are you?" she said at the beginning of the first visit. Climbing the stairs was when she felt most breathless and most anxious.

Intervention over four home visits with CBIS physiotherapist included:

- Education on genesis of breathlessness and anxiety cycle.
- Advised not to become obsessive monitoring oxygen saturations.
- Demonstrated than Mrs Jones may still feel breathless with good oxygen saturations i.e. effort of breathing, not always low oxygen levels, causing breathlessness.
- Positioning at rest to aid relaxation of breathing accessory muscles.
- Home exercise programme on DVD, while using ambulatory oxygen as prescribed.

- Practiced exercises with clinician, who gave advice on maintaining moderate breathlessness during exercise
- Paced breathing with exercise using pursed-lips breathing, lengthen out breath and breathing out on effort, use of fan, recovery breathing and positioning post exercise to aid recovery. (Due to severe emphysema and very hyperinflated lungs found Breathing Control very difficult therefore focused on other breathing techniques).
- Inspiratory muscle training with prolonged out breath after inspiration to avoid breath stacking.

Visit	SOB at rest	Anxiety at rest	SOB climbing stairs	Anxiety climbing stairs
11th Sept (First visit)	3	3	10	7
27th Nov (Final visit)	2	0	5	0

SOB (shortness of breath) & anxiety measured using the modified Borg score.

Referred onto community respiratory team for continued home exercise with the aim of attending Pulmonary Rehabilitation in the future. Mrs Jones's long-term goal was to leave her scooter outside a shop and browse shop with daughter.

A Selection of Exercise and Activity Opportunities

Home exercise programmes: Written, DVD, online, interactive games console. Home exercise equipment-bike, rower, treadmill etc.

Traditional exercise: Gym, exercise classes, swimming, aqua fit, cycle riding.

Sports and activities: Dance, bowls, table tennis, badminton, bowling, archery, rowing, golf.

Walking: Walking for Health group often based at health centres, Ramblers association walks, pedometer/ step counter walking programme, Nordic walking (walking with two poles to improve trunk and upper limb training), dog walking for friend or animal shelter if don't own a dog.
Gym Referral Scheme: Patients with specific medical conditions may be entitled to reduced cost gym scheme lead by an instructor with training in long term medical conditions. A referral to the scheme from their GP or other medical professional is usually required.
Personal Health Coach: Patients with specific medical conditions may be entitled to a specified number of sessions with a personal health coach who may advise on exercise, diet and smoking cessation.
Tai Chi: Slow movement routines and static postures encouraging relaxation and gentle breathing. May help to improve balance.
Yoga: Sustained postures often involving gentle stretching, balance and postural stability combined with slow, deep breathing and relaxation. Slow, deep breathing may not suit patients with obstructive airways disease as may increase hyperinflation.
Pilates: Gentle exercise to improve muscle tone, posture and core stability.
Exercise for the over 50s or those with chronic conditions: Groups often available at local leisure centres or community centres. May run traditional classes at a low intensity and with the specific needs of this group in mind. May also offer other leisure activities at a reduced cost such as bowls, badminton, dance, Tai Chi etc.
Inspiratory muscle training (**IMT**): Devices provide inspiratory resistance with the aim of strengthening inspiratory breathing muscles.
Neuromuscular electrical stimulation (**NMES**): Provides electrical stimulation to skeletal muscles causing regular contractions with the aim to improve their strength.

Pedometer (Step Counter) Walking Programme

"*Made me realise how little exercise I was doing*"
"*A useful incentive to make me go out for a walk*"
"*I could build up my walking gradually, without 'over doing it*"
A selection of patient comments regarding using the 'step counter' pedometer

Walking daily or on most days after pulmonary rehabilitation has been shown to slow the decline in health related quality of life as well as slowing the progression of breathlessness experienced during daily activities (Heppner et al. 2006).

Maintaining regular physical activity is key to breathlessness self management in long term conditions, yet this can be very hard to achieve.

A step counter is a very basic pedometer, it simply counts the number of steps a person takes rather than calculating distances and calories burned etc. They are inexpensive, easy to obtain, simple to use and do not require any information to be inputted when set up. They can be worn hung around the neck, hidden under clothing or clipped onto a belt or waist band. The step counter must remain up-right so the weight inside can 'jog' up and down to in time with the patient's steps and therefore count them. For this reason patients with large waists or loose waist bands may find a neck worn step counter may be more accurate.

Traditional Step Counter Walking Programme

- Wear the step counter all day, every day, from when you get dressed until you get ready for bed.

- Record the daily step count and re-set the counter each evening to zero.
- **First week**: Just record the daily step count. Do not try to increase the number of steps.
- **Week 2**: Take the average daily step count from week one and add 10 % or 500 steps to this average. This becomes the new daily step count goal.
- **Weeks 3 and beyond**: Repeat week 2 and set a new daily step count goal based on previous week's daily average plus 10 % or 500 steps.

If the mathematics is too complicated then just ask the patient to try to ensure that their weekly step total is higher than the previous week.

Be Active Ltd (2009)

The daily number of steps when 'well' may provide a baseline of activity which can then be used as a 'bench mark' to build up to following an exacerbation, hospital admission or treatment, such as chemotherapy.

For patients with very low exercise tolerance the step counter can be used to monitor and encourage walking within the home and maybe combined with a goal such as 'to walk the length of the house every hour' or 'to take two walks a day around the garden'.

For the anxious patient worried about walking outdoors and becoming 'stranded' by breathlessness or fatigue the patient may ask a relative to walk the intended outdoor distance with the step counter and record the number of steps. The patient then uses this number of steps as a goal. The patient can wear the step counter and gradually build up to walking this number of steps, stopping to rest or use breathlessness management techniques as required, in the 'safety' of the home and garden before walking the distance in public, perhaps with a relative or friend the first time.

An alternative walking programme that does not involve a pedometer or step counter is suggested by the British Lung Foundation and can be found on their website.

Case Study: Walking Programme

Mr Smith, 63 year old gentleman with COPD. Has done Pulmonary Rehabilitation in the past but declined to repeat it as he says he does not like group work. Finds home exercise boring and therefore reduced motivation to do these. Enjoys walking out doors but lacks confidence as he fears his breathlessness will become uncontrolled and he won't be able to walk back home. He has not been out much during the winter due to cold weather and his breathlessness has become worse as a result.

Seen for three home visits over a period of 6 weeks. Intervention included:

- Explained the deconditioning cycle and importance of maintaining strength and fitness to help with managing breathlessness.
- Anxiety cycle and discussing fears regarding breathlessness becoming out of control.
- Breathing control at rest and when walking. Paced breathing with walking including lengthening out breath and pursed-lips breathing.
- Use of a walking stick to use as a 'portable leaning post' when out walking and identifying places to stop and rest along walk i.e. Seats to sit on and fences to lean on.
- Used step counter to count steps walking around garden and how often need to stop and rest (initially with clinician then alone).
- Translate number of steps when walking in garden to walking short distances down road and back (initially with clinician then alone).
- Gradually increased walking distance outdoors as confidence increased.

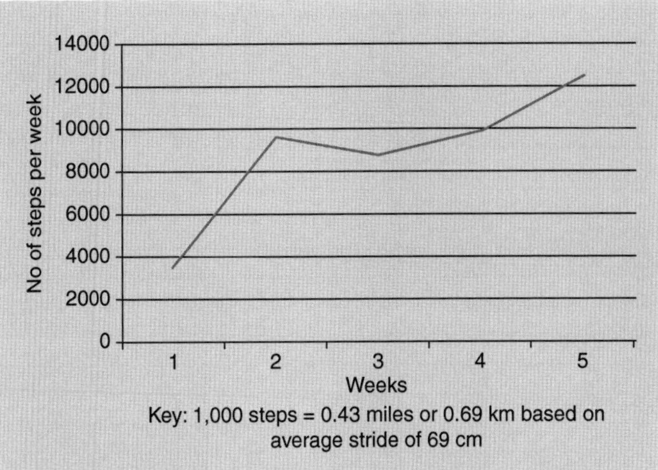

Mr Smith no longer fears his breathlessness will become uncontrolled as he has confidence in the strategies to manage it. He is able walk around his local park, sitting to rest on benches or leaning on his stick as required and can walk to walk to a nearby bus stop. He continues to use his pedometer to maintain his daily walking distance and to gradually build up his exercise tolerance after an exacerbation of COPD.

Step 6: Ongoing Motivation

Maintaining motivation can be the hardest step in exercise and activity promotion. In the long-term patients need to be self motivators with regard to exercise and activity. They need to understand that it is a life time commitment and therefore not an easy task. Ultimately the exercise or activity must be enjoyable and achieve the patient's goals to ensure long-term motivation. Patients need to realise that exacerbations of their condition will reduce their physical fitness and this may affect their motivation however they should not give up. Steel et al. (2010) showed that COPD patients who complete pulmonary rehabilitation with an interruption due to exacerbation still made similar gains to those who completed the programme without interruption.

Maintaining Motivation

- Ensure the exercise or activity is fun and enjoyable
- Record exercise progress
- Set and review SMART goals
- Reward achievement
- Modify exercise to suit the patient's needs as well as to maintain interest
- Make exercise and activity a social occasion by going with friends or relatives.
- Ensure the patient has a realistic plan of long term exercise or activity post completion of pulmonary rehabilitation or other short term exercise programme
- Following an exacerbation or relapse of the chronic condition a review and support to improve exercise and activity levels is recommended

Summary

"*The magnitude of the effect of pulmonary rehabilitation on* ***exercise capacity, dyspnoea and health related quality of life*** *are significantly greater than the effects of bronchodilator drugs*" – Consensus statement, National Clinical Guideline Centre 2010 p.264

Maintaining exercise and activity levels are key in the long-term management of breathlessness. It is therefore the role of all clinicians working with breathless patients with long-term conditions to ensure exercise and activity, linked to patient goals, is promoted at every opportunity, to help maintain motivation to exercise and remain active at all stages of the patient's life.

Key Points

- Explore and address the patient's barriers to exercise.
- Discuss and address any fears the carer may have regarding their loved one becoming breathless on exertion.
- Ensure patient and carer understand that breathlessness in its self is not harmful. Becoming breathless is a normal response to exercise and will actually help to improve cardiovascular health
- Discuss and set SMART patient orientated goals.
- Agree on an exercise or activity routine that is enjoyable, feasible and appropriate.
- Monitor progress, progress exercise or activity and set new goals.
- Encourage patient to reward achievement.

References

American College of Sports Medicine (ACSM). American College of Sports Medicine roundtable on exercise guidelines for cancer survivors. Med Sci Sports Exerc. 2010;42(7):1409–26.

American Thoracic Society & European Respiratory Society (ATS/ ERS). American Thoracic Society and European Respiratory Society statement on pulmonary rehabilitation. Am J Respir Crit Care Med. 2006;173: 1390–413.

Be Active Ltd. Pedometer walking programme advice leaflet. 2009. www.be-activeltd.co.uk.

Benton MJ, Swan PD. Addition of resistance training to pulmonary rehabilitation programme: an evidence-based rational ad guidelines for use of resistance training with elderly patients with COPD. Cardiopulm Phys Ther J. 2006;17(4):127–33.

Borg GA. Psychophysiological bases of perceived exertion. Med Sci Sports Exerc. 1982;14:377–81.

British Thoracic Society (BTS) & Association of Chartered Physiotherapists in Respiratory Care (ACPRC). Guidelines for the physiotherapy management of the adult, medical, spontaneously breathing patient. Thorax. 2009;64(I):i1–51.

British Thoracic Society (BTS) & Scottish Intercollegiate Guidelines Network (SIGN). 101 British guideline on the management of asthma: a national clinical guideline. 2012. www.brit-thoracic.org.uk.

Campbell A, Foster J, Stevinson C, Cavill N. The importance of physical activity for people living with and beyond cancer: a concise evidence review. London: Macmillan Cancer Support; 2012. http://www.macmillan.org.uk/Documents/AboutUs/Commissioners/Physicalactivityevidencereview.pdf.

Celli BR. Exercise in the rehabilitation of patients with respiratory disease. In: Hodgkin JE, Celli BR, Connors GL, editors. Pulmonary rehabilitation: guidelines to success. 4th ed. St Louis: Mosby Elsevier; 2009. p. 129–42.

Department of Health. Start active, stay active: a report on physical activity from the four home countries chief medical officers. London. 2011.

England R, Maddocks M, Manderson C, Wilcock A. Factors influencing exercise performance in thoracic cancer. Respir Med. 2012;106(2):294–9.

Evans RA, Singh SJ, Morgan MD. A randomised controlled trial of pulmonary rehabilitation for patients with chronic heart failure. Eur Respir J. 2007;28(S50):766s.

Gosselink R, De Vos J, van den Heuvel SP, Segers J, Decramer M, Kwakkel G. Impact of inspiratory muscle training in patients with COPD: what is the evidence? Eur Respir J. 2011;37(2):416–25.

Heppner PS, Morgan C, Kaplan RM, Ries AL. Regular walking and long-term maintenance of outcomes after pulmonary rehabilitation. J Cardiopulm Rehabil. 2006;26(1):44–53.

Morris GS, Gallagher GH, Baxter MF, Brueilly KE, Scheetz JS, Amhed MM, Shannon VR. Pulmonary rehabilitation improves functional status in oncology patients. Arch Phy Med Rehabil. 2009;90(5):837–41.

National Clinical Guideline Centre. Chronic obstructive pulmonary disease: management of chronic obstructive pulmonary disease in adults in primary and secondary care. London: National Clinical Guideline Centre; 2010. Available at http://guidance.nice.org.uk/CG101/Guidance/pdf/English.

National Institute for Health and Clinical Excellence (NICE). Idiopathic pulmonary fibrosis: the diagnosis and management of suspected idiopathic pulmonary fibrosis. NICE clinical guideline 163. 2013. www.nice.org.uk.

National Institute for Health and Clinical Excellence (NICE). Chronic heart failure: management of chronic heart failure in adults in primary and secondary care. NICE clinical guideline 108. 2010. www.nice.org.uk.

O'Shea SD, Taylor NF, Paratz J. Peripheral muscle strength training in COPD: a systematic review. Chest. 2004;126:903–14.

Puente-Maestu L, Sanx ML, Sanx P, et al. Comparison of effects of a supervised vs self monitored training programme in patients with chronic obstructive pulmonary disease. Eur Respir J. 2000;15(3): 517–25.

Speck R, Courneya K, Masse L, Duval S, Schmitz K. An update of controlled physical activity trials in cancer survivors: a systematic review. J Cancer Surviv. 2010;4:87–100.

Spence RR, Heesch KC, Brown WJ. Exercise and cancer rehabilitation: a systematic review. Cancer Treat Rev. 2010;36:185–94.

Steel BG, Belza B, Cain K, Coppersmith J, Howard J, Lakshminarayan S, Haselkorn J. The impact of chronic obstructive pulmonary disease exacerbation on pulmonary rehabilitation participation and functional outcomes. J Cardiopulm Rehabil. 2010;30(1):53–60.

Further Information & Resources

Walking groups and Pedometers

Be Active Ltd. Official distributers of the walking for health step counters (pedometers). 2013. www.be-activeltd.co.uk.

British Heart Foundation. Walking training schedules. 2012. http://www.bhf.org.uk/get-involved/events/training-zone/walking-training-zone/walking-training-schedules.aspx.

Walking for health. 2013. www.walkingforhealth.org.uk.

Exercise and COPD

BLF Exercise Instructors. 2013. http://www.blf.org.uk/Page/Respiratory-exercise.

British Lung Foundation (BLF). Exercise handbook. BLF: London; 2011. http://www.blf.org.uk/Page/Exercise-Handbook.

Asthma and Exercise

Asthma UK. Living with asthma: exercise. 2012. http://www.asthma.org.uk/knowledge-bank-living-with-asthma-exercise.

Physical Activity and Cardiac Disease

British Heart Foundation. Get active, stay active. 2012. http://www.bhf.org.uk/publications/view-publication.aspx?ps=1001248.

British Heart Foundation. Physical activity and your heart. 2013. http://www.bhf.org.uk/publications/view-publication.aspx?ps=1001061.

Exercise and Activity for People Living with and Beyond Cancer

Macmillan Cancer Support. Move more: physical activity the underrated 'wonder drug'. 2012. http://www.macmillan.org.uk/Documents/Cancerinfo/Physicalactivity/Physicalactivitycampaignreportlores.pdf.

Macmillan Cancer Support. Move more patient information pack. 2012. http://www.macmillan.org.uk/Documents/Cancerinfo/Physicalactivity/movemore.pdf.

Self Management of Long Term Conditions

Expert Patients Programme Community Interest Company. Self management in long-term health conditions: a handbook for people with chronic disease. Boulder: Bull Publishing Company; 2007.

Chapter 9
Supporting Carers

Evidence

There are a number of studies which explore the lived experience of being a carer (McNamara and Rosenwax 2010; Currow et al. 2008; Curt et al. 2000). This important data provide healthcare professionals with valuable insights into what it is like to live with a patient experiencing the consequences of a long term or progressive illness with symptoms like breathlessness. Booth et al. (2003) discovered that carers of breathless patients suffer physically and psycho-socially in a different way to patients, but with equal severity. Evidence to support the effectiveness of specific interventions to improve the quality of life for carers is sparse but this is an emerging field of research. (Vernooij-Dassen et al. 2011) reviewed cognitive reframing interventions, which are intended to reduce carer stress by changing their beliefs and perceptions regarding their roles and responsibilities as carers. They found that these had a possible impact on reducing stress, anxiety and depression in carers of people with dementia. Other studies have shown that interventions for people experiencing breathlessness have had a subsequent favourable effect for carers also (Farquhar et al. 2010). Candy et al. (2011) also reviewed the evidence for supporting carers of patients in the terminal phase of disease. They found that "supportive interventions" may reduce

S. Booth et al., *Managing Breathlessness in Clinical Practice*, DOI 10.1007/978-1-4471-4754-1_9,

psychological distress and improve quality of life but recommended further research to understand better any specific benefits on physical health and well-being and to elucidate the interventions of benefit for carers.

Introduction

> He says he can't breathe but he has enough air to yell at me
> It's terrible to see it.........and you feel so helpless, so useless, so useless, I don't know how you can help really
> (Booth et al. 2003)

It is easy for clinicians to focus exclusively on the person experiencing breathlessness, inadvertently overlooking the impact on the carer or loved one(s) and how they feel about witnessing this distressing symptom. It can be as frightening to watch someone in the grip of an episode of breathlessness as it is to experience it personally. This is particularly true if the carer has no idea what to do to manage it, which can lead to a sense of helplessness or futility. Breathlessness can be extremely upsetting to experience, and to watch this can evoke exactly the same emotions, often coupled with a sense of helplessness if the individual is unable to reduce the impact on their relative.

As well as having to observe someone they are caring for experience breathlessness on a regular basis, there are a number of other factors specific to being a carer which need to be considered. Carers of those with advanced cardio respiratory disease are often over the age of 60 and have their own health problems. Many will already have a caring role for children, grandchildren and/or elderly parents. Often reluctant to express or address their own needs and feeling a need to put the patient first, it is common for carers to relinquish their own work roles to care for their loved one, which will invariably have a financial and social effect on them as individuals. As well as a change in working role, the carer may also have lost social contacts with friends and acquaintances due to the increasing demands on their time. By the same token, many hobbies or interests may have had to be resigned.

On the other hand, caring for someone can be a very positive experience and one which brings people together, sharing time and activities that they have not previously had the opportunity or inclination to do. Caring for someone who is breathless, regardless of whether this is a positive experience or not is usually very tiring and the carer will often describe feelings of fatigue and even exhaustion.

It is vital to consider how to support the carer as part of any effective self-management programme or intervention for breathlessness as they are a **key** component in how the person will manage this symptom.

To help us understand some of the specific issues for carers, it is helpful to look at these in relation to the breathing, thinking, functioning (BFT) model outlined in Chap. 1.

Case Study

Mrs Orange is a 62 years old lady. She has been married for 44 years and she and her husband have three children and seven grandchildren, whom she provides child care for to enable her daughters to continue to work part-time. Mrs Orange has recently taken on the caring role for her husband, who was diagnosed with COPD 3 years ago. He is becoming more breathless and, as a result, she prefers him to stay at home and rest, which has meant that the household and gardening tasks that would usually be carried out by her husband now fall to her. Mrs Orange did used to have a part-time job as a receptionist in the local GP practice, a role which she thoroughly enjoyed, but has had to resign due to the increasing demands on her time with caring for her husband. She is terrified by his breathlessness, and although she does not want him to go to hospital, feels reassured when she calls for an ambulance as they are able to relieve his breathlessness. She does try to encourage him to take big breaths, to try and get more air in when he is breathless, but he just gets cross, and snaps at her, which makes her feel even more desperate. He doesn't like the grandchildren coming round any more, what used to be fun, now feels so stressful.

Breathing

We have discussed patients' misperceptions of needing to take big breath in to "get more air" and the same misunderstanding could equally be applicable to carers. Upon seeing their loved one becoming increasingly breathless and distressed, carers can often give well-meaning advice, such as "take a big breath" or "big breaths in" in an attempt to help when this only exacerbates the problem. There may also be a tendency to draw upon personal experiences, such as being in labour or breathing control for sporting activities.

Thinking

Often carers will describe feelings of frustration, anger, worry, anxiety, distress or guilt. Indeed sometimes they may be feeling these emotions but for many reasons be unable or reluctant to express them.

Negative Emotions

Frustration

Caring for someone experiencing breathlessness can be incredibly frustrating as it often places limitations or significantly alters usual activities and routines. Carers may be unable to carry out the things that they enjoy because of the constraints imposed by their partner's condition. They may also become frustrated about not knowing what to do either for the patient, the patient's condition or to manage their own mental and physical wellbeing.

Anger

Most models of grief incorporate a period of anger, and with the likelihood of having many losses to contend with when living with someone experiencing breathlessness (loss of the routines, shared activities, the person they know as their partner) it is not surprising that carers may feel a certain level of anger at some point. These feelings of anger may manifest in many ways and may also be aimed at the patient, healthcare professionals, others around or themselves…Carers may occasionally feel bitter; about what has happened to them in life, about what they may see as the self-inflicted nature of the relative's illness or about the lack of help they perceive they get from the NHS or from friends or society in general. Anger, if aimed at the person they are caring for, may also be reciprocated, which can result in an uncomfortable and unhappy situation needing sensitive and careful handling in order to suggest any helpful strategies to manage

Anxiety and Worry

To witness someone who is breathless can be extremely anxiety provoking. Carers can often feel very anxious and frightened about their relative's breathlessness, particularly if they feel they cannot influence this or do anything to improve it. Carers may share common thoughts with patients such as fearing that the person is going to stop breathing. Excessive worry can lead to anxiety and depression and it is important for the carer to be encouraged to seek an assessment of their own health if this is the case. It is not uncommon for carers to become clinically depressed; to have feelings of worthlessness, guilty ruminations and obtaining no pleasure from life. Carers may well have a health condition of their own and may also feel worried that they have to sacrifice their own self-management to care for their loved one experiencing breathlessness. Changes to employment, regarding them or their partner, resulting in financial difficulties, may also contribute to these feelings of worry and stress. Carers can also feel torn between the various commitments on their time, such as having other family members to care for or wishing to spend time away from the home or their loved one but worrying how they will be whilst left alone.

Distress

Carers may also be distressed by the state that their relative is in, often describing being mentally "torn apart" by watching somebody breathless. A perception of helplessness in the situation or the fact that they do not feel they do enough can also cause distress or feelings of exasperation.

Guilt

Guilt is another common feeling experienced by carers and one which is difficult to alley. There are many reasons given for these feelings of guilt; feeling guilty for not caring enough, feeling guilty for not doing enough, feelings of not meeting expectations of them as a career, comparisons to others who they perceive as doing "much better" given the same situation. Ironically, strategies employed to enable carers to have respite from their situation often leave them with feelings of guilt for leaving their loved one, even if this helps the overall situation in the long run.

Positive Emotions

Pride

Carers may well feel proud of what they are doing and rightly so. Often they may feel that no-one else can do the job as well as they are doing, which may well be a challenge when discussing or suggesting the involvement of paid carers. Carers may feel that empowered and undoubtedly have particular knowledge and insight into how their relative is feeling or what they are experiencing. A certain sense of pride in the way they are looking after the person, and how they are managing a difficult situation may also be present as well as feeling proud of the way they manage or co-ordinate services that care for their spouse or relative.

Self-Efficacy

Caring for a loved one can evoke a sense of self-efficacy, perhaps satisfaction having mastered the intricacies of the medical system and the NHS. They may also feel a greater sense of achievement in what they have learned from looking after their relative and enjoy acting as their advocate.

Functioning

Social isolation and loneliness are common consequences, particularly when caring over many years, and may carers may have noticed a reduction in their engagement in enjoyable activities and hobbies. Much time may be expended on caring routines, leaving little time for hobbies and social contacts. Although carers often increase their "workload" and tasks within the home, they may well spend less time on their own fitness or health, such as not being able to attend the gym or walk out as much, which can result in them becoming de-conditioned in addition to the patient. Carers often feel completely exhausted because they are not only carrying out their own tasks of everyday living but also all the things that used to be done by their relative and in addition may be giving physical care to their loved one.

Strategies to Support Carers

Breathing

It is vital that the carer understands the basic mechanics of breathing and the importance of efficient breathing to enable them to encourage and reinforce these principles at times when the patient is breathless. Practising breathing control techniques with the carer themselves trying the exercises can also be beneficial in helping them to experience the desired efficient breathing.

Thinking

Many carers find great reassurance in the fact that breathlessness in itself is not harmful and will recover using appropriate techniques. In the midst of a breathlessness episode, it is often the carer who is first at hand to reassure the patient, so armed with correct information and knowledge; they can make an enormous difference in the outcome of such an episode.

It is also worth taking some time to consider what the carer's thinking process is and what impact this is having on them directly. Addressing any misperceptions, such as worrying about the patient stopping breathing or dying "gasping for breath" can be useful in alleviating anxiety and worry.

Functioning

Principles of energy conservation, such as activity pacing, planning, prioritising and engaging in meaningful activities and exercise are equally applicable to carers as well as patients. It is important to acknowledge how exhausting caring is, both physically and mentally, and give the carer "permission" to express this.

Action Plans / Ritual for Crises

Action plans or a "ritual for crises", providing a strategy to manage breathlessness episodes, can be helpful for carers as well as patients. Agreeing a plan which is personalised to the individual and carer, can be a useful strategy. It can act as a vital prompt or reminder to reduce feelings of anxiety or panic in the midst of a breathlessness episode. Laminating such a plan for the carer to have to hand when needed may even prevent the need to call for additional help or emergency services.

Recognition and Acknowledgement

So much emphasis is given to the person experiencing breathlessness, and time limitations often result in the needs of the carer being inadvertently overlooked. Treating the career as an individual and acknowledging and addressing their own needs can be enormously beneficial in recognising their role and the impact that it is having on them. They are not simply an extension of the caring team and should not be assumed to be there simply to soak up as much knowledge as possible about their relative's illness and then carry out allotted tasks for keeping that person out of hospital or to spare the clinical team's effort.

Respecting Autonomy

Carers may wish to carry out some tasks to enable the patient to manage their breathlessness live with their condition with as much autonomy as possible and to be as well they can, but equally they may wish to minimise their input into clinical matters. Respecting their wishes and being careful not to place any expectation on them to carry out caring duties can help them to maintain their own health and well-being.

Support

To support, as far as possible, the carer to have a life of their own, albeit in a different way to that they lived previously, enabling them to have some time free from caring to enjoy activities which are most important to them. In order to do this you need to find out what those activities are.

To give the carer the opportunity to be supported in their own way whilst respecting the patient's wishes. For example, while the patient may not wish to talk about their illness or any fears regarding the future, carers may need to do this frequently. They may wish to express grief or fear or tears, and may need "permission" to feel comfortable to do so.

Respite

Although respite care is very rarely available on an in-patient basis, other options can be explored to provide the carer with respite from their situation. Alternative forms of respite may include private carers coming into the home so that the patient does not have to have their routine disrupted very much (often a source of great anxiety) thus allowing the carer to go away, perhaps stay with other family members or take a holiday. Volunteer groups can also sometimes provide cover for a day or afternoon. The carer may benefit from a carers assessment carried out by social services or an organisation such as Crossroads Care. If symptom control issues exist it may be possible to admit the patient for symptom control to a local hospice before the carer becomes completely exhausted and distraught.

Differing Priorities

When meeting with patients experiencing breathlessness and their careers, it may often become apparent that their priorities and goals are vastly different. Focussing on acknowledging these differences and setting achievable goals can be a starting point to negotiate agreed goals that both parties are happy with (Table 9.1).

> It has helped her, which is the important thing...my wife's been, not necessarily sorted, but understanding what she can and can't do better.....it takes a lot of stress and worry away from us
>
> As a family it has [helped], because we all now understand better the problem that she's had. So we can adapt our lives, our way of living more so around my wife to compensate.....to help her
>
> (Booth et al. 2003)

Summary

Carers individual needs are often overlooked resulting in them getting insufficient support and attention. In the worst scenario, this can have a significant impact on their own health and wellbeing and threaten the sustainability of the patient's care. Funding constraints often result in no specific services for carers being commissioned which results in this support often being sought from voluntary services. Support for and involvement of the carer in the management of breathlessness is vital and can be fundamental in the successful management of this symptom. For Mrs Orange, it would be important to listen to her experience of being a career of someone experiencing breathlessness and acknowledge the compromises that she has had to make. Further exploration around her feelings of being "terrified" when she witnesses the breathlessness and addressing any misperceptions would be useful. It would also be helpful to go through breathing control techniques as a more helpful strategy than trying to encourage "deep breaths" which should be discouraged. Advice regarding the benefits of engagement in exercise for Mr Orange would be helpful and may even enable them to regain some activities that they previously enjoyed together,

Table 9.1 Practical strategies to support carers

Area of support	**Possible suggestions**
High quality patient care	Optimisation of the patient's health significantly helps the carer as well as the patient. Creating effective out of hours support is of particular value.
Clinical support	Repeat prescriptions delivered to the home, organised transport to appointments and home visits can greatly reduce the demands on the carer.
Self-help groups	Local support groups, on-line discussions forums and help lines provided by charitable organisations can be very helpful in providing social and peer support as well as practical advice and information
Befriending services	Befriending throughout the illness trajectory, often by volunteers, appears to lead to a reduced need for subsequent bereavement support
Family and psychological support services	Burdens placed on carers can put strain on marital and family relationships, leading to unhappiness and tension at home. Referring on to appropriate services can reduce the likelihood of this occurring.
Primary health care teams.	The carers' health must be attended to, particularly as it is common for elderly carers to have their own medical conditions
Home carers	Carers can come from statutory social services, private sources and charities; It is helpful to encourage carers to use the time for recreation, rather than practical tasks.
Respite care	Some residential or nursing homes provide respite care but this is rarely free. Hospice and other day centres can also give carers valuable hours of respite
Financial Support	This is often needed, particularly when carers have had to leave paid employment. Carers may be entitled to a range of benefits as well as flexible employment opportunities.

perhaps even involving the grandchildren. Any action plans would need joint agreement but there is scope for a number of strategies to be employed to improve Mrs Orange's quality of life.

Key Points

- Caring for a person experiencing breathlessness can be exhausting and stressful
- Acknowledging a carer's individual needs is important
- Carers will often need "permission" to express their own thoughts / emotions and needs
- Education for the carer is fundamental to successful self-management of breathlessness
- Reducing carer anxiety can lead to better coping strategies and may reduce the need for the patient to require emergency hospital admissions

References

Booth S, Silverster S, Todd C. Breathlessness in cancer and chronic obstructive pulmonary disease: using a qualitative approach to describe the experience of patients and carers. Palliat Suppor Care. 2003;1:337–44.

Candy B, Jones L, Drake R, Leurent B, King M. (2011) Interventions for supporting informal caregivers of patients in the terminal phase of a disease. Cochrane Database Syst Rev. (6):CD007617.

Currow D, Ward A, Clark K, Burns C, Abernathy A. Caregivers for people with end-stage lung disease: characteristics and unmet needs in the whole population. Int J Chron Obstruct Pulmon Dis. 2008;3(4): 753–62.

Curt GA, Breitbart W, Cella D, Groopman JE, Horning SJ, Itri LM, Johnson DH, Miaskowski C, Scherr SL, Portenoy RK, Vogelzang NJ. Impact of cancer-related fatigue on the lives of patients: new findings from the fatigue coalition. Oncologist. 2000;5:353–60.

Farquhar M, Higginson IJ, Fagan P, Booth S. Results of a pilot investigation into a complex intervention for breathlessness in advanced chronic obstructive pulmonary disease (COPD): brief report. Palliat Support Care. 2010;8:143–9.

McNamara B, Rosenwax L. Which carers of family members at the end of life need more support from health services and why? Soc Sci Med. 2010;70:1035–41.

Vernooij-Dassen M, Draskovic I, McCleery J, Downs M. (2011) Cognitive reframing for carers of people with dementia (Review). Cochrane Database Syst Rev. (11):CD005318.

Part V
An Integrated Strategy

Chapter 10
Pharmacological Management of Breathlessness

It is clear that breathlessness has many neurophysiological similarities to pain – both are

- integrated in the central nervous system
- comprise qualitatively distinct sensations
- modulated by signals from the 'higher' areas of the CNS, cortical regions where thinking, feeling and previous experience can exacerbate or palliate the sensation
- influenced by outputs from the limbic system: anxiety and other unpleasant affective states can increase the severity of these symptoms.

There are, however, major differences in the pharmacological management of pain and breathlessness. Drug treatment for malignant pain has progressed enormously in the last 20 years. There is an expectation that patients with uncomplicated pain from cancer will have excellent control on oral drug therapy alone, often a combination of drugs working in different ways. Only 5–10 % of patients with intractable or complex pain will require anaesthetic, radiological or very rarely surgical interventions (as attempts to get the best relief possible) and still continue to have significant pain. Although improvement is possible with current drug therapy, sadly clinicians cannot reassure patients that any medicines taken specifically to improve breathlessness will achieve excellent relief, returning the patient to a state in

S. Booth et al., *Managing Breathlessness in Clinical Practice*, DOI 10.1007/978-1-4471-4754-1_10,

which they are free of the symptom and as active as before. The evidence base, although improving is also thinner.

Another difference from pain, is that the same management strategies are presented as appropriate for both malignant and non-malignant breathlessness. It is not confirmed that there is a final common pathway for breathlessness of all aetiologies, though it seems likely, so we currently consider pharmacological treatment for both sorts of breathlessness as the same, with prognosis and severity the guides to when and what sort of drug therapy should be initiated. In contrast, there are marked differences in the management of malignant and non-malignant pain which are considered almost as separate entities. Palliative care physicians are rarely involved in the management of stable, chronic non-malignant pain in those with years to live; anaesthetists usually lead the multiprofessional teams which care for these patients. Drugs, anaesthetic, surgical and radiological interventions are seen to be of limited in value in chronic non-malignant pain in if not used in conjunction with behavioural and psychosocial approaches.

Slowly Progressive or Rapidly Progressive Breathlessness

> The division into malignant and non-malignant breathlessness does not correlate with the patient's lived experience, patients with some non-malignant diseases can have very rapid, frightening deteriorations in their breathlessness. It is more accurate to consider breathlessness as *slowly* or *rapidly progressive*.

Patients with chronic non-malignant breathlessness from COPD and those with lung cancer have different disease trajectories (outlined in Chap. 1) but there are more indolent cancers where patients live with breathlessness for many years. Some patients with fibrosing lung disease experience rapidly progressive 'malignant' breathlessness with a concomitant physical and social decline.

> The individual patient's prognosis is central to the decision about which drugs are used, by which route, and when they are initiated to palliate breathlessness.

For many patients, especially these with chronic intractable breathlessness who are mobile and who may live with it for years, rather than months or weeks, drug treatment is a second choice, and non-pharmacological, (also known within CBIS as pro-central) interventions remain the most appropriate management strategy.

In this chapter, those drugs routinely used in breathless patients are considered individually and their use in patients discussed in those (1) breathless on exertion (2) breathless on minimal exertion, such as talking, hair brushing, washing or dressing (3) breathless at rest, i.e. continuously even without exertion (4) breathless and entering the end of life phase.

Drugs are discussed in order of the depth of the evidence base available for each one, and those which are used rarely or experimentally are only briefly reviewed.

> It is sometimes justifiable to use a drug for which there is little evidence, to try to help a patient in desperate suffering, at the end of their life, provided you have a rationale. Using a drug with a poor evidence base should be done after discussion with a specialist with experience in this area, most commonly a palliative care physician.

Individual Drugs

Opioids e.g. Morphine, Fentanyl, Hydromorphone, Buprenorphine, Diamorphine

Opioids have the best evidence base of all the drugs used in the management of breathlessness. Most of the (small number) of trials carried out have been done using morphine sulphate immediate release solution and morphine sulphate modified release tablets such as MST. The earliest evidence was a systematic review carried out by Jennings et al. (2002), which has never been repeated. Then a fully powered RCT was carried out in medical in-patients (most of whom had COPD) by Abernethy et al. (2003), and there have been other studies since looking at dosing regimens and safety. To date most trials have used opioids for days to weeks or at most 3 months, longer is needed to establish safety and acceptability when prescribing a drug that may be used for years in moderately breathless patients with COPD. There is a relatively high attrition rate in those using opioids for breathlessness, mostly attributed by participants to adverse effects of the drugs.

Possible Mechanisms of Action

The areas of the brain concerned with the genesis of breathlessness are particularly rich in mu receptors which are found throughout the CNS and the respiratory system. Morphine and other opioids form a family of drugs which primarily stimulate the mu receptor. This underlies the rationale for using them in breathlessness, though their use originally followed from clinical observation and physiological evidence – it had been shown that opioids reduced the rate and increased the tidal volume of respiration.

Opioids

1. reduce the drive to breath and the discomfort of air hunger, rather than reducing the sensation of called 'the work of breathing.' The reduction in respiratory drive reduces corollary discharge (see page 19)
2. modulate cortical activity reducing the sensation of breathlessness
3. reduce the anxiety associated with breathlessness
4. may act through causing sedation, even if not overt
5. there is a postulated effect on the production of endogenous opioids (β endorphins) which bind to opioid receptors
6. have an effect on peripheral opioid receptors in the lung

> There is a growing evidence base demonstrating that opioids are helpful in the palliation of the intractable breathlessness associated with advanced disease.

Indications

Whilst most clinicians have little hesitation in using opioids in breathless patients with cancer who have months to live there is still sometimes a reluctance to use them in patients with COPD. However important international guidelines for the management of this symptom (e.g. GOLD) in COPD have begun to recommend opioids for these patients.

Patients with interstitial lung disease (ILD) are often tachypnoeic with an increased work of breathing: opioids may be particularly helpful in this situation.

Using Opioids to Palliate Breathlessness

Patients Breathless on Exertion

In these patients most clinicians would prefer to use a physically rehabilitative approach first backed up by non-pharmacological, procentral approaches to aid motivation and concordance. This is the approach that CBIS uses. Of course there are grades of severity of 'breathless on exertion:' some patients who describe themselves as very troubled by breathlessness can walk substantial distances (e.g. a mile or more) others who use the same sort of description can only one flight of stairs or walk 100 yards before they have to stop. In those who border on 'breathlessness on slightest exertion' an approach that combines a reversal of deconditioning, other procentral approaches and then possibly opioids may be most helpful. These patients, intuitively, may also be particularly helped by walking aids or neuro-muscular electrical stimulation to help 'kickstart' their rehabilitation.

If these approaches have been tried, with appropriate support, and not been helpful or been unacceptable then treatment with an opioid may be helpful (using the regimen discussed below) but it is in this group that the adverse effects of opioids are most likely to lead to the rejection of this treatment.

Patients Breathless on Minimal Exertion

> This group of individuals may live for years with breathlessness suffering greatly and opioids can play an important part in providing relief for these patients – pro-central and rehabilitative non-pharmacological approaches should also be used.

At CBIS we use a regimen of slow titration of opioid and we always discuss the prescription with the respiratory clinician (or other specialist) caring for that patient as well as the family doctor. Some patients with COPD go into Type II respiratory failure during exacerbations and it is essential that this group stop opioid use during these times, unless monitored in hospital. Sometimes other clinicians, unfamiliar with the use of opioids in breathlessness may take the initiation of opioids as a sign that the patient is entering the end of life phase, such misunderstandings or worse, the stopping and starting of opoids with conflicting messages from different caring teams is very detrimental to a patient's morale and trust in those teams. This is best avoided by excellent communication. The respiratory specialists and others involved in that patient's care need to support the prescription. A co-ordinated approach to opioid prescription is essential.

The starting dose of opoids on this regimen is low enough that those patients may not notice any change in their breathlessness initially. We use this regimen:

1. To avoid sedation or other adverse side effects, like nausea, which may discourage the patient from using opioids and which are less likely with a "start low and increase slow" *regimen.*
2. To avoid respiratory depression in patients, particularly those with CO_2 retention, where it is difficult to monitor a patient in the community.
3. In order to reassure other clinicians not used to giving opioids to patients with non-malignant disease.
4. Many patients with advanced non-malignant disease and breathlessness have lived with the symptom for months, even years. Opioids are going to make possibly a 20 % impact on the patients' breathlessness at best. Rapid titration is more likely to lead to adverse effects and the patient may lose the willingness to use the drugs at all. Other clinicians unused to using opioids in non-malignant disease may be deterred from using them if they get unfavourable feedback. A slow titration, that may take some weeks to get maximum benefit, may be better both strategically and clinically. Opioids are a precious evidence-based drug, it is important not to alienate patients by adverse effects. Slow titration is used for drugs used in other conditions to minimise adverse effects e.g. antidepressants for neuropathic pain.
5. It is easier to find the **lowest** effective opioid dose. Most people would prefer to be on the lowest dose of a drug possible.

Opioid titration in non-malignant disease in the community by CBIS protocol

Daily dose	A.M.	P.M.
Week 1	1 mg Oramorph®	Nil
Week 2	1 mg Oramorph®	1 mg Oramorph®
Week 3	2 mg Oramorph®	1 mg Oramorph®
Week 4	2 mg Oramorph®	2 mg Oramorph®
Week 5	5 mg modified release	Nil
Week 6	5 mg modified release	Up to 1 mg Oramorph®
Week 7	5 mg modified release	Up to 2 mg Oramorph®
Week 8	5 mg modified release	Up to 3 mg Oramorph®
Week 9	5 mg modified release	up to 4 mg Oramorph®
Week 10	5 mg modified release	5 mg modified release. Formal review by GP

1. At each stage decide whether you need to increase the dose or whether it can remain the same.
2. May decide to decrease to "last effective dose"; increase not always needed.
3. There is no "right" dose; the dose is what is best for the patient.
4. Dose needs review preferably weekly by District Nurse/GP/Community Matron.
5. Consider using alternative opioids.
6. Can use buprenorphine patches. Start with 5 µg per hour patch.

Reproduced with permission from 'The Breathlessness Intervention Manual' (2012)

An Alternative View

There are two schools of thought on using opioids for breathlessness in non-malignant disease. The CBIS approach is outlined above and is also used by Graeme

Rocker in Canada. Amy Abernethy, David Currow and others use opioids from the start in higher doses, such as 10 mg of modified release morphine daily and titrate upwards. CBIS uses a more rapid regimen in some individuals, e.g. those in hospital, those with cancer (e.g. some patients with ILD) and it is likely that different conditions will need different opioid titration. Most studies have not found doses above 20 mg MR morphine per day necessary. Those few pharmacovigilance studies which exist have found no evidence of respiratory depression. **Watch the evidence in this area**.

Patients Breathless at Rest

This group are likely to benefit from opioids and receive less benefit from other non-pharmacological approaches. They find it harder to participate in exercise though facilitating physical and mental activity remains important for their overall health. The fan, energy conservation, and breathing retraining can still be used with great benefit. NMES may prove particularly helpful in this group. Opoids may make it possible for such patients to be more active and a virtuous circle of some improvement ensue. We recommend the same regimen in this group.

Patients who are breathless at rest have a poor prognosis and it is important to initiate discussions about future goals and patients' wishes for the sort of care they want, when they do enter the end of life phase to be started at this point, if not previously attempted.

Patients Entering or Line the End of Life Phase

Many will want improvement in their symptoms with the least degree of sedation possible.

The pharmacological management of this phase is discussed in detail in Chap. 11. The priority at the end of life is for the patients to be comfortable; there is no anxiety about long-term adverse effects or dependency. The only caveat is that the patients must be involved in the discussion, they may not wish to risk any sedation or they may actively want sedation. A commonly used combination in the last days or sometimes weeks of life is a subcutaneous infusion of diamorphine (UK only) or morphine or other soluble opioid and midazolam. Occasionally levomepromazine or haloperidol may be used with an opioid.

Cautions

Opioids should be used with caution, i.e. with advice from a specialist in their use the following situations

1. **In those patients with CO_2 retention or those who have CO_2 retention during exacerbations.** As opioids reduce the drive to breathe (part of their mechanism of action in relieving breathlessness) they can cause dangerous respiratory depression in those who already have a flattened respiratory response to CO_2.
2. **In those with a history of substance abuse**: these patient should not be denied pharmacological relief of their breathlessness but a particular regimen may be needed the patient themselves may refuse to use them (fearing a return to dependency) or they may live in a community where another drug is preferable
3. **In those with renal failure**: such people can have opioids but morphine is not ideal as it has active metabolites and the excretion of these is reduced in renal impairment leading to an unpredictably long half life. An oral prn ('as needed') regimen should in theory, not cause problems (as if the patient is drowsy they simply will not take the drug) but most clinicians would use an alternative opioids not dependent on renal excretion (such as alfentail) in these circumstances, even though it has to be given parenterally. If there is no other drug available and the patient is at the end of life, using morphine intermittently, titrated against response, may be the right thing to do. Discussion with the patient is essential.

Most of the time morphine is the drug of choice particularly because of its flexibility to be used as a small oral dose (immediate release) and a modified releases preparation. Some experts avoid the use of fentanyl patches as this drug reaches higher than normal blood levels in the presence of acidaemia, as it is displaced from its protein binding. Acidaemia is relatively common in chronic advanced COPD particularly during exacerbations or when the patient is unwell for other reasons. The absorption of fentanyl through the skin is increased when patients are vasodilated and this occurs in hypercarbia (raised arterial CO_2) a worsening cycle of increasing Type II respiratory failure can occur. Fentanyl which delivers a fixed dose regimen with a long period after the patch is removed before blood levels fall to zero is probably best avoided in managing breathlessness.

Route of Administration

Until the end of life phase, (or in the presence of nausea and vomiting or went the oral route is simply not available) morphine should be given by mouth either as solution, immediate release or modified release tablet. Buprenorphine may be used as a topical preparation.

Adverse Effects

Opioids have well recognised adverse effects, it is common for patients to develop tolerance to some of these (e.g. sedation, if titration is slow) and not to others (e.g. constipation).

The adverse effects of morphine include:

- **Nausea and vomiting**: this is very common and can be reduced by careful titration, use of prophylactic antiemetics in those prone to nausea or early use (having them in the house before starting the morphine) of these drugs. Morphine both slows gastric emptying and causes nausea by stimulation of the chemoreceptor trigger zone in the brain stem. Commonly used antiemetics include low dose haloperidol (1.5–3.0 mg daily in divided doses) or metoclopramide (typically 10 mg orally tds).

- **Sedation**: this too is very common when the drug is initiated or the doses increased. It can be reduced by slow titration but if persistent, a change in the opioid used may be indicated. Many patients fear sedation and it may discourage patients from continuing these drugs if they experience it early on.
- **Constipation**. Again this is common and aperients need to be started when morphine is, a stimulant and softener in combination is necessary. Some commonly used in palliative care when the prognosis is limited (co-danthrusate) are contraindicated in long-term use. There is huge inter-individual variation in the severity of constipation so careful drug titration is necessary, severe constipating is very exhausting for a breathless patient and it is essential to avoid this.
- **Fear of morphine**. Morphine is still a feared drug and associated with the end of life by many patients or their families and by some clinicians. It is essential to invest the time in talking to patients (and their families) before it is used to ensure that any concerns are aired and reassurance given where it can be. Talking to colleagues unused to using morphine for breathlessness can also prevent problems.
- **Respiratory depression**. Opioids palliate breathlessness partially through respiratory depression but careful titration should ensure that dangerous respiratory depression is avoided. Discuss the reduction or cessation (temporarily) of opioids during an exacerbation with the respiratory clinician treating the patient if there is any doubt about whether the patient has or develops Type II respiratory failure.
- **There is now discussion in the literature about the safety of opioids in the longer term in those patients with a life expectancy of months to years.** There are clearly changes in the blood oxygenation and respiratory pattern of patients with normal lungs on opioids for treating non-malignant pain and this should raise questions about the use of opioids in the long term in those with a longer prognosis

Chronic Non-malignant Versus Malignant Disease

An approach to chronicity is discussed in the final chapter but the use of a drug over years which has only been scientifically tested in patients over months is never satisfactory. Consider non-pharmacological treatments first in those patients who have breathlessness on exertion, may live for years and can engage in self-management programme. Even in the pharmacovigilance studies published, only one in three patients derive benefit at 3 months and many stop taking opioids because of adverse effects.

Benzodiazepines

Benzodiazepines, notably lorazepam and midazolam, are commonly prescribed in palliative care patients for the management of breathlessness. In fact, there is very little evidence for their effectiveness, although it is fair to say that there is very little research in this area. Simon et al. 2010, conducted a Cochrane review of the available trials in the use of Benzodiazepines in breathlessness and found only seven trials to review, even these were methodologically flawed and concluded that 'benzodiazepines should be used in the pharmacological management of breathlessness only after opoids and other approaches had been tried. '

There was some data, from a study in dying patients, to suggest that opoids and benzodiazepines used together may have some synergy. These drugs are commonly used in this way at the end of life.

> Apart from the end of life phase or if there is otherwise unmanageable anxiety, when short term use of days may be indicated) benzodiazepines should not be used for breathlessness in those who have a prognosis of years

What Are the Problems with Benzodiazepines?

1. High level of dependency – patients can easily become dependent on these and will have an extremely difficult time withdrawing them, with a recrudescence of anxiety amounting to terror being very common. Diazepam was widely used in the 1970s as a general anxiolytic and there are still people suffering today with flashbacks from difficulty coming off diazepam.
2. Sedation, benzodiazepines can cause significant drowsiness and prevents the user from driving or operating machinery. Driving is often of central importance to breathless patients for maintaining some sort of independence.
3. The number needed to treat (NNT) is greater than the number needed to harm in the elderly with possible cumulation leading to increased risk of falls

Drug Portraits

Lorazepam: a drug with a moderately long half life (16 h) which is commonly used 'pro re rata' (PRN or 'as needed) for patients with intrusive anxiety. Given sub-lingually it has a rapid onset of action being absorbed through the wall of the vessels under the tongue directly into the blood stream.

Diazepam: has a very long half life and active metabolites (desmethyldiazepam) and can have a cumulative half life in the hundreds of hours. It is not recommended.

Midazolam is a water-soluble benzodiazepine that does have a short half life of 4–5 h but it has to be given intravenously or subcutaneously it is most commonly used by the latter route in patients at the end of their lives.

Mirtazapine

There is great interest in this drug which is a pre-synaptic alpha2-adrenoceptor antagonist i.e. it inhibits α 2 adrenergic, 5-HT2 and 5HT3. Serotinergic pathways and receptors are known to be involved in the genesis of breathlessness and it is thought that antidepressants acting on the serotinergic pathway may modify central cortical perception of breathlessness as well as acting at brain stem level.

It was noted that breathlessness could be reduced with the use of SSRIs (selective serotonin reuptake inhibitors), even when patients were not distressed or very anxious. . In patients with advanced disease SSRIs are often contraindicated because of the number of potential drug interactions in this group of people who often take many drugs.

Mirtazapine has found favour with clinicians because

- It is better tolerated than the SSRIs with fewer adverse effects such as early anxiety and nausea and vomiting
- It is anxiolytic and improves sleep at lower doses being slightly sedating and prescribed at night
- It has a faster onset of action that SSRIs (1–2 weeks) in depression
- It has good efficacy for depression in many patient groups including those with cancer
- It is available in a number of formulations (15 and 45 mg tablets, oro-dispersible and liquid formulations).
- The dosing regimen is simple and well understood.

The sedative effect at lower doses is due to the antihistaminergic effects predominating; at higher doses there is an increased noradrenergic effect.

Possible adverse effects include;

- Somnolence
- Weight gain
- Increased appetite

If not distressing to the patient, these can be useful. Sleep is often disturbed in breathless patients, they are often anxious and patients with advanced disease have often lost weight.

Indications

There are no firm indications for mirtazapine yet as it has not been formally tested for its use in breathlessness but using the available evidencc mirtazapinc is worth trying

1. Certainly when a patient is depressed and breathless
2. When pharmacological intervention is indicated but the patients does not want or has stopped using opoids
3. When there is sleep disturbance
4. When there is anxiety.

It is always worth explaining that mirtazapine is an antidepressant (even if the patient is not depressed) and giving a rationale for its use based on its modulation of central perception. If a patient finds out from the internet, or a friend or relative that is an antidepressant and you have not told them this, it can lead to mistrust.

Other Psychoactive Drugs

Many of the drugs that affect breathlessness are centrally acting, and most are psycho active. There is limited data on the following which should be used only after discussion with a specialist.

Phenothiazines – there is a minimal amount of evidence to suggest that phenothiazines may be helpful in breathlessness. They are also, however; drugs with wide-ranging pharmacological effects, including hypotension because of alpha-adreno receptor activity. They may be helpful when terror or severe anxiety, which cannot be addressed in any other way, is a prominent symptom, and they are very appropriate at the end of life, e.g. levomepromazine is often used at this time.

Buspirone is not chemically related to barbiturates or other sedative or anxiolytic drugs. Its prime use is as an anxiolytic agent in mental health. There has long been interest in his drug but all the clinical trials so far completed in patients with malignant and non-malignant breathlessness have failed to show any impact on the symptom when compared with placebo.

Other drugs that have been used, for which there are small trials available, include furosemide, nabilone and other cannabinoids.

Furosemide causes bronchodilation and this explains the rationale for its use, the theory seems to be stronger than the practice as several trials have failed to show any benefit but these have been small and further investigation is needed.

The case report and studies reporting benefit have all been carried out in patients with cancer and breathlessness, towards the end of life when other treatment has failed. The drug has been given by nebuliser. It is probably best used after discussion with a specialist.

There is emerging evidence that nebulised opioids and furosemide may be useful in certain patients with breathlessness. It is well established that there are opioid receptors in the lung and that furosemide is a bronchodilator so there are continuing trials.

Keep watching the evidence.

Key Points

- In a patient who is comfortably mobile and has a long prognosis, concentrate on non-pharmacological interventions
- In a patient who is breathless at rest, be ready and willing to prescribe opioids, even early in treating the cause
- In a patient who is breathless on the slightest exertion, or on exertion, consider opioids
- In a patient who is at the end of life, use sub-cutaneous opioids and benzodiazepines by continuous infusion and PRN as needed for comfort
- Consider mirtazepine in a depressed patient, however breathless, in an anxious patient or one who does not want for use morphine, or who is sleeping badly.

References

Abernethy AP, Currow DC, Frith P, Fazekas BS, McHugh A, Bui C. Randomised, double blind, placebo controlled crossover trial of sustained release morphine for the management of refractory dyspnoea. BMJ. 2003;327(7414):523–8.

Jennings AL, Davies AN, Higgins JP, Gibbs JS, Broadley KE. A systematic review of the use of opioids in the management of dyspnoea. Thorax. 2002;57(11):939–44.

Simon ST, Higginson IJ, Booth S, Harding R, Bausewein C. Benzodiazepines for the relief of breathlessness in advanced malignant and non-malignant diseases in adults (Review). 2010. The Cochrane Collaboration. Published by JohnWiley & Sons, Ltd.

Further Reading

Booth S, Bausewein C, Higginson I, Moosavi SH. Pharmacological treatment of refractory breathlessness. Expert Rev Respir Med. 2009; 3(1):21–36.

Currow DC, McDonald C, Oaten S, Kenny B, Allcroft P, Frith P, Briffa M, Johson MJ, Abernethy AP. Once-daily opioids for chronic dyspnea: a dose increment and pharmacovigilance study. J Pain Symptom Manage. 2011;42(3):388–99.

Davenport PW, Vovk A. Cortical and subcortical central neural pathways in respiratory sensations. Respir Physiol Neurobiol. 2009; 167(1):72–86.

Johnson MJ, Abernethy AP, Currow DC. Gaps in the evidence base of opioids for refractory breathlessness. A future work plan? J Pain Symptom Manage. 2012;43(3):614–24.

Mahler DA. Opioids for refractory dyspnea. Expert Rev Respir Med. 2013;7(2):123–35.

Rocker G, Young J, Donahue M, Farquhar M, Simpson C. Perspectives of patients, family caregivers and physicians about the use of opioids for refractory dyspnea in advanced chronic obstructive pulmonary disease. CMAJ. 2012;184(9):E497–504.

Chapter 11
Care Towards the End of Life for the Breathless Patient

Twelve principles of a good death (Debate of the Age Health and Care Study Group 1999**)**

- To know when death is coming, and to understand what can be expected
- To be able to retain control of what happens
- To be afforded dignity and privacy
- To have control over pain relief and other symptom control
- To have choice and control over where death occurs
- To have access to information and expertise of whatever kind is necessary
- To have access to any spiritual or emotional support required
- To have access to hospice care in any location
- To have control over who is present and who shares the end
- To be able to issue advance decisions which ensure wishes are respected
- To have time to say goodbye, and control over other aspects of timings
- To be able to leave when it is time to go, and not to have life prolonged pointlessly.

S. Booth et al., *Managing Breathlessness in Clinical Practice*,
DOI 10.1007/978-1-4471-4754-1_11,

Introduction

> There is evidence that the degree of breathlessness is a more reliable indicator of a poor prognosis than disease severity or pulmonary function. Breathlessness has also been shown to be a risk factor for emergency room attendance, hospital admission and readmission, and for in-hospital death (Nishimura et al. 2002; Steer et al. 2011).

Breathlessness is undoubtedly a frightening symptom; patients tend to intuitively understand its adverse prognostic significance. Reaching the end of life is no less so; fear of the unknown and distress at the prospect of leaving close family is inevitable. It is therefore not surprising that, for patients, carers and professionals, coping with breathlessness towards the end of life is particularly challenging.

A number of studies have identified patients' priorities towards the end of life. Consistent findings are that patients wish to be given as much control as possible, to have time to prepare for death and to retain dignity. Each of these principles relies on understanding that the prognosis is poor and communicating openly within families and with professionals. However, prognostication can be difficult, especially in advanced non-malignant respiratory disease, with its unpredictable disease trajectory. This, therefore, is a core challenge when caring for breathless patients towards the end of life. Without an understanding that the end of life is approaching, good care cannot be achieved.

Symptom control can also be a challenge. A self-management approach, emphasised throughout this book as the most effective ways of managing breathlessness, becomes difficult in far advanced disease. It is not easy for patients to learn new techniques, and only those already known and practised are likely to be useful. Deep terror can result from the prospect of dying breathless, with patients and their families naturally imagining 'dying gasping for breath', 'suffocating at the end' and 'horrifying panic'. Furthermore, family carers, at a time when their support is particularly vital, are often already deeply exhausted with no further reserves of resilience.

Most patients wish to die out of hospital. Indeed, when asked in advance, less than 5 % would choose to die in hospital. In reality, however, over 50 % of patients are hospitalised at the very end of life and, in patients with advanced non-malignant respiratory disease, the figure is substantially higher. Hospital deaths may not be well-managed, in an environment designed to provide acute care, and the majority of hospital complaints relate to poor end of life care. Uncontrolled symptoms, fear, carer exhaustion and, above all, a failure to predict impending death, are all factors that lead to emergency hospital admission and inadequate care.

Mr Jones was a 78 year old farmer with advanced COPD. He had had four hospital admissions already over the last year, each time with an infective exacerbation of COPD and a step-wise deterioration in condition. He had been house-bound between admissions, and was rarely able to leave the sitting room of his bungalow where he slept in a chair.

He arrived in hospital by ambulance, drowsy and agitated, accompanied by his wife. He had another chest infection, his GP having started antibiotics in the community 3 days earlier. There had been no improvement in his condition and he was now clearly in respiratory failure. He was commenced on non-invasive ventilation (NIV), and became increasingly agitated, attempting to remove the mask.

His condition continued to deteriorate and the admitting team decided that the 'ceiling of care' should be intravenous antibiotics and NIV. When the junior doctor explained that he was very unwell and they wanted him to be 'not for resuscitation', his wife became extremely distressed, shouting "Why are you giving up on him now? He has always got better before." She tried to insist that he must go to ITU and be resuscitated, but felt that she was being ignored. He died a few hours later, with the NIV mask still strapped on. His wife was devastated and, a few days later, registered a formal complaint about his care.

Despite the challenges, the premise of this chapter is that it *is* possible to provide excellent care at the end of life for breathless patients. Central to this is the process of advance care planning, with early and open communication giving patients the time to plan and take control. Careful symptom control, good psychological care and support for carers are also vital component of good end of life care.

Care for those approaching the end of life cannot be, and indeed should not be, simply the domain of palliative care specialists. All healthcare professionals should be able to provide good quality generalist palliative care for their patients. The relative neglect of end of life care until recently may be due, in part, to death being viewed as a failure in medical care, rather than inevitable. It is a duty and privilege to be able to provide compassionate and effective care from diagnosis to death (Spathis and Booth 2008).

Open Communication

Talking about dying does not bring it any closer. It is about making plans so that you can make the very best of living.

How could Mr. Jones' traumatic death have been avoided? Mr Jones was too unwell to have decision-making capacity, and his wife clearly did not understand his poor prognosis. In the crisis of his final admission, she interpreted 'not for resuscitation' as 'not for active treatment', and understandably felt confused, abandoned and distressed. The crises was, sadly, almost inevitable. It could only have been avoided if, at an earlier stage, there had been an opportunity for sensitive, open discussion about his prognosis. Mr Jones could have been encouraged to express his views about his future care. His wife's role in the last few days of his life would then have changed from a devastated bystander to the person caring for him in the way he chose. After his death, she could have been fulfilled from knowing she had cared for him in the way he had wanted.

Advance care planning is a voluntary process of discussion about future care, between patients, carers and professionals, which occurs in anticipation of a potential loss of decision-making capacity. It includes:

- Developing a shared understanding of the illness and prognosis
- Understanding the patients' values and personal goals of care, and
- Eliciting patients' specific preferences in terms of treatments and place of care.

Evidence

Research

- Advance care planning increases patient and family satisfaction with care, and reduces carer stress, anxiety and depression (Detering et al. 2010).
- Open conversations enhance rather than diminish hope (Davison and Simpson 2006). This may be because the hope is now realistic and focused on achievable goals.
- End of life discussions lead to less aggressive care, with an associated improvement in quality of life (Wright et al. 2008).

- Nurses supported to undertake advance care planning conversations experience greater job satisfaction and feel empowered to provide appropriate care (Seal 2007).
- The vast majority of patients attending pulmonary rehabilitation would welcome the opportunity to talk openly and plan their future care (Burge et al. 2013; Heffner et al. 1996).

Public surveys

- 60–70 % of patients are comfortable talking about dying but most professionals think patients are not.
- Less than 5 % of patients initiate a discussion about end of life choices with their GP, but 90 % continue a conversation initiated by the GP.
- Most people (60–70 %) fear lack of choice about where they die, and lack of open conversations.

Barriers

Despite the evidence for potential benefit from open communication, it is equally clear that these conversations do not often happen, particularly in the context of advanced non-malignant disease such as COPD and heart failure.

The main barrier is prognostic uncertainty which can lead to so-called 'prognostic paralysis'. The possibility of the prognosis being longer than expected may hinder open communication about it being potentially short. It can be argued, conversely, that the possibility of the prognosis being short should drive early attempts at communicating more openly. In practice, it is human nature to try to avoid potentially emotive conversations, unless absolutely necessary. The societal and cultural taboos in relation to talking about dying are well recognised and, in the UK, the national Dying Matters coalition (www.dyingmatters.org) is making progress is breaking down these barriers at a societal level.

Other barriers include health carers' fear of upsetting patients or reducing hope which, from the evidence above, can be seen to be an unnecessary concern. Patients, in turn, do not want to upset the professionals, perhaps fearing that they are implying a failure on their part. Patients also have an erroneous expectation that clinicians will initiate the conversation. Furthermore, patients may choose to deny a poor prognosis, and may feel that care planning is therefore irrelevant.

Practical Tips

Healthcare professionals tend to be over-optimistic in their attempts to prognosticate. Consider trying the following:

- Ask the 'surprise question': 'Would I be surprised if this patient was to do in the next few months?' If the answer is 'no', it may be time to try to discuss prognosis and care planning.
- In malignant disease, assess the rate at which the patient's condition is changes. If deterioration is obvious month by month, the prognosis may be measured in months; if week by week, in weeks; and if day by day, in days.
- Assess performance status. Patients who spend more than 50 % of waking time lying down tend to have a prognosis of less than 3 months.
- Consider the severity of breathlessness. There is evidence that the degree of dyspnoea is a reliable indicator of both a poor prognosis and a willingness to discuss end of life issues.

When talking about prognosis the following tips may be helpful:

- Avoid being too specific, and talk in terms of 'many months', 'weeks to months', 'days to a few weeks' and so on. Patients receiving a quantified prognosis tend to anticipate the expected date with dread, hindering their ability to live as well as possible until they die.
- Acknowledge the inherent uncertainty, and introduce the concept of 'making parallel plans' or 'hoping for the best,

preparing for the worst'. This process of 'parallel planning' tends to be highly acceptable to patients, allowing a discussion about a potentially poor prognosis, in the context of retaining hope for a better outcome.

Triggers for open conversations in breathless patients who may be approaching the end of life include the following:

- Indicators of a potentially short prognosis (see above)
- Multiple recent hospital admissions
- Patient cues, such as expressing worry about the future, or fear about burdening family
- Particular distress or frustration, suggesting a mismatch between understanding and reality
- Commencing a significant new treatment such as NIV, second line chemotherapy etc.

Advance care planning usually involves a series of conversations, and views may change over time. Try to establish patients' overall views about how aggressively they wish to be treated in the future, as well as more specifically their opinion about specific treatments, and where and by whom they would like to be cared for.

One specific treatment is cardiopulmonary resuscitation (CPR) in the event of a cardiorespiratory arrest. CPR is highly unlikely to be helpful in patients who are breathless from advanced, progressive disease. It is important to avoid patients becoming burdened by being asked to make a decision about CPR, when it would in fact be futile.

- Remember that conversations about CPR in this context are often a compassionate explanation of a clinical decision, rather than a consultation

- The priority is for advance care planning to occur, with an understanding of the prognosis, and a discussion about those treatments that *would* be helpful
- It is worth proactively addressing common misconceptions. 'Not for CPR' does not mean 'not for active treatment'.

Useful phrases include:

- 'It is often easier to talk through decisions when there isn't a crisis'
- 'Have you thought about the type of care you would like if you were ever too sick to speak for yourself?'
- '... helping you stay in control'
- 'We are hoping that your next chest infection will respond to antibiotics like this one did. However, we are very bad at predicting the future. Some patients find it helpful to hope for the best, while at the same time planning for the 'what ifs'...

Avoid the phrases 'there is nothing more we can do' or 'withdrawing treatment'.

Healthcare is provided by a multitude of teams across a range of settings. There is no value in having these important conversations, if the outcome is not communicated clearly. A number of methods have been developed, ranging from a clinical letter copied to all key members of the wider healthcare team to, more recently, electronic databases incorporating advance care planning information and accessible from all settings.

Some patients simply do not want to talk openly about the future. It is vital *never* to push a patient in such situations; advance care planning is absolutely not a 'tick box' exercise. Denial is a reasonable coping mechanism and should never be forcibly countered. However, sometimes if it is proving difficult to engage patients in open conversation, consider suggesting to them that you want to help them stay in control and avoid future crises. Patients with advanced disease tend to feel out of control (which is true in terms of the disease progression), and relish any prospect of controlling at least some aspects of their life. Patients also tend to respond to the idea of 'supporting or unburdening their family' by avoiding putting family members in a future position of perceiving they are making decisions for the patient.

When patients prefer not to talk openly or if a conversation is not feasible, for example if there is no time or during a medical crisis, it is worth making contact with an appropriate professional who knows the patient well in their usual place of care (in the UK, this may be the patient's general practitioner or clinical nurse specialist). Such an individual may then try to explore the patient's wishes at a later date. This may be directly with the patient or, with the patient's consent, with a relative or carer who may have an understanding of the patient's views and goals for care.

Symptom Control

It is impossible to achieve a 'good death' without good symptom control. Many patients, and indeed professionals, fear that palliation of breathlessness will be hard to achieve at the end of life. In practice, however, breathlessness tends to become less severe in the last days of life for a number of reasons:

- Activity reduces as people spend more time in bed, and therefore the demand on the respiratory system falls.
- There has been time to adjust to the short prognosis and, with acceptance, distress tends to diminish.
- In type 2 respiratory failure, accumulating carbon dioxide tends to cause drowsiness and a sense of calm.

It is important to elicit patients concerns about symptom control towards the end of life. Once they have admitted their fears ('Will I die gasping for breath?'), any misconceptions can be addressed. The sense of relief is usually considerable when patients realise that their fears, although understandable, are unfounded.

Practical Tips to Manage Breathlessness and Anxiety

In the last few weeks and days of life, symptom palliation requires a move from predominantly self-management (non-pharmacological) techniques to the use of drug therapy. Self-management techniques that have been taught and practiced at an earlier stage can, however, be usefully continued and may include the following:

- Careful positioning (see page 44)
- Use of a handheld fan or small room fan, propped close to a patient's face if too weak to hold
- Relaxed breathing (see page 193)
- Relaxation techniques, particularly guided imagery.

Pharmacological approaches include use of the following: (Booth 2009)

- Low dose opioids, usually oral morphine or subcutaneous morphine/diamorphine (see page 34)
- Benzodiazepines, often sublingual lorazepam or subcutaneous midazolam
- Other anxiolytic drugs, such as mirtazipine (orally) or levomepromazine (orally or subcutaneously).

Oxygen rarely has a place in the palliation of breathlessness in the last days of life (see page 37)

> In the last days of life, effective symptom palliation can be achieved by setting up low dose morphine/diamorphine and midazolam in a syringe driver. In an opioid naive patient, consider using morphine or diamorphine 2.5–5 mg/24 h and midazolam 5 mg/24 h as a starting dose. This can be titrated upwards carefully according to clinical need. Small 'as needed' doses should also be prescribed, such as morphine or diamorphine 1.25–2.5 mg

sc prn, and midazolam 2.5 mg sc prn or lorazepam 0.5 mg sublingual prn. In patients already taking strong opioids for pain or breathlessness, an equivalent dose subcutaneous infusion can be set up, titrating the dose according to individual need.

Practical Tips to Manage Other Symptoms

Once patients become too weak to cough, retained secretions can lead to noisy respiration which may be upsetting for family and, indeed, professionals to hear. It is believed however not to distress the patient, and explanation of this alone, can often ameliorate family anxiety. Repositioning of patients into a semi-prone position can be helpful. Parenteral antisecretory drugs such glycopyrronium and hysocine butylbromide are often used, although this practice is not evidence-based, and these drugs can cause a dry mouth and uncomfortable thickening of chest secretions.

Cough, pain and agitation may all occur, and are managed pharmacologically with the same drugs that palliate breathlessness, low dose opioids and benzodiazepines. Whereas at an earlier stage, encouragement of expectoration and sputum thinning approaches are helpful, at the very end of life, cough suppression is usually necessary.

A degree of dehydration is physiological towards the very end of life. Patients naturally drink less. Indeed, full hydration at a time of organ failure and poor membrane function can be counterproductive, with fluid accumulation (such as pulmonary oedema, pleural effusions, peripheral oedema) contributing to poor symptom control. This can be an important point to explain to family members, as misconceptions can arise that contribute to family distress.

Breathless patients who mouth breathe tend to suffer from a dry mouth towards the end life. A dry mouth is uncomfortable and also appears to reduce the effectiveness of the fan in palliating breathlessness. Careful attention to good mouth care is important. Consider the following:

- Stopping inappropriate oxygen and anti-secretory drugs, which dry the mouth and are usually ineffective in symptom palliation
- Treating oral candidiasis, which is a particular problem in patients on steroids
- Debriding a furred tongue with a soft toothbrush or placing a quarter ascorbic acid tablet on the tongue
- Smearing paraffin ointment on the lips
- Encouraging regular sips of cold water or carbonated lemonade, or sucking of ice chips
- Considering regular use of artificial saliva sprays.

Carer Support

The unmet needs of carers are increasingly recognised, and support of this key group of people is described in detail in chapter 9. Towards the end of life, carer suffering may be compounded. Carers may not understand or accept the poor prognosis. Carers may have little experience of witnessing dying and, particularly in the context of breathlessness, may be fearful of how they will cope. Anxiety, sadness and a sense of helplessness are predominant emotions, and physical exhaustion after a long illness can compound the emotional turmoil. Carers often focus on the needs of the patient, to the detriment of their own.

There are a number of ways of supporting carers of breathless patients towards the end of life:

- Early encouragement of open communication is particularly helpful for family members. If a patient does not want to talk, he or she may still give consent for family to talk with health care professionals.
- Compassionate acknowledgement of the carer's predicament and innate resilience can be enormously empowering.

- Practical support is inevitably appreciated, ranging from equipment, such as a hospital bed, to arranging carers, organising respite care and providing support with financial matters. Try to involve appropriate services, such as a community palliative care team, as early as possible, so that the patient and carers have time to adjust to new relationships.

Key Points

"Despair is most often the off-spring of ill-preparedness"
Don Williams Jr

- A 'good death' can only be achieved with *early* communication and planning, acknowledging a short prognosis and giving the patient control over how the last part of his or her life is lived.
- Parallel planning is an important concept when caring for breathless patients with an uncertain prognosis towards the end of life.
- Most patients would prefer to die at home. This can only be achieved with careful planning, anticipation of future problems, excellent symptom control and strong carer support.

L was a 43 year old medical secretary diagnosed 3 years ago with a metastatic osteosarcoma. She 'fought' as hard as she could, insisting on further lines of chemotherapy each time her disease relapsed. In the last few months of her life, she became increasingly breathless, with a huge burden of pulmonary metastatic disease. As she became more breathless, her fears compounded, and she became increasingly vociferous in her complaints about the care she was receiving. She refused to discuss her prognosis or her future, each time threatening, 'Don't you dare give up on me'.

She was eventually admitted to hospital with a chest infection, having been deteriorating despite oral antibiotics at home. During her first night in hospital, the ward nurse was setting up her intravenous antibiotics, when she broke down in tears. 'What is going to happen now? I am so frightened…' The nurse stopped her work, sat down and listened carefully. Slowly at first, L began to talk about her fears. A torrent of concerns followed, central to which was the estrangement from her father back in Scotland.

Talking openly now about her poor prognosis, she begged to be given intravenous antibiotics until 'she could sort things out'. Over a series of emotional telephone conversations, she made progress in resolving an old dispute and a range of family conflicts. The ward teams noted her increasing calmness, and improved symptom control, even though objectively her clinical condition was worsening.

L chose to go home to spend the last few days of her life with her husband and dogs. The night before she was discharged, she called the ward nurse to her bedside. "It is so strange. Only when I accepted I was dying did I truly start living… I should have done this earlier, but I am so grateful for every day of living that I have left."

References

Booth S. End of life care for the breathless patient. Gen Pract. 2009;39–43.

Burge A, Lee A, Nicholes A, et al. Advance care planning education in pulmonary rehabilitation: a qualitative study exploring participant perspectives. Palliat Med. 2013;27(6):508–15.

Davison S, Simpson C. Hope and advance care planning in patients with end stage renal disease: qualitative interview study. Br Med J. 2006;333(7574):886. doi:10.1136/bmj.38965.626250.55.

Debate of the Age Health and Care Study Group. The future of health and care of older people: the best is yet to come. London: Age Concern; 1999.

Detering K, Hancock A, Reade M, Silvester W. The impact of advance care planning on end of life care in elderly patient: randomised controlled trial. Br Med J. 2010;340:c1345. doi:10.1136/bmj.c1345.

Heffner JE, Fahy B, Hilling L, et al. Attitudes regarding advance directives among patients in pulmonary rehabilitation. Am J Respir Crit Care Med. 1996;154:1735–40.

Nishimura K, Izumi R, Tsukino M, Oga T. Dyspnoea is a better predictor of 5-year survival than airway obstruction in patients with COPD. Chest. 2002;121(5):1434–40.

Seal M. Patient advocacy and advance care planning in the acute hospital setting. Aust J Adv Nurs. 2007;24(4):29–36.

Spathis A, Booth S. End of life care in chronic obstructive pulmonary disease: in search of a good death. Int J Chron Obstruct Pulmon Dis. 2008;3(1):11–29.

Steer J, Norman E, Afolabi O, Gibson G, Bourke S. Dsypnoea severity and pneumonia as predictors of in-hospital mortality and early readmission in acute exacerbations of COPD. Thorax. 2011;67(2):117–21.

Wright A, Zhang B, Ray A, et al. Associations between end of life discussions, patient mental health, medical care near death, and caregiver bereavement adjustment. JAMA. 2008;300(14):1665–73.

Chapter 12
An Approach to the Breathless Patient

"I was thrilled to bits to be able to be getting some knowledge of what my complaint was all about..."

pt participating in Booth et al. (2003), p. 293

This chapter sets out an approach to helping the breathless patient (and their family) by synthesising the practices discussed in this book and integrating them with current best practice. Indicative work from laboratory studies and from those other specialities which care for patients with chronic disease.

It will already be clear that a system for giving the best care to a person suffering from the chronic, intractable breathlessness of advanced disease, cannot be contained within a set of algorithms to be delivered in a fixed order.

Individual assessment is essential followed by the instigation of a strategy, decided with the patient, using evidence-based practice, to help reduce the impact of breathlessness and the suffering it causes, and addressing the more general difficulties of living with any chronic condition.

Breathlessness is very complex, and this complexity increases with chronicity. If the patient cannot find a way to manage their breathlessness (and the other burdens of chronic illness) and receives no effective help, life can become desperate. The impact of chronic breathlessness infiltrates every aspect of a person's existence and profoundly

S. Booth et al., *Managing Breathlessness in Clinical Practice*,
DOI 10.1007/978-1-4471-4754-1_12,

affects those closest to them. Rather than a simple uni-dimensional sensation which can be switched off by one intervention it is an experience of the mind and body. Cicely Saunders, founder of the modern specialty of palliative care, described 'total pain' which had spiritual, psychological, social as well as physical aspects and this concept can also be used for breathlessness.

The complexity of chronic breathlessness is one of the reasons that it is so difficult to treat and possibly explains why research in this area was overlooked for so long.

Using the Research Evidence

Evidence from outside breathlessness research can help clinicians to give patients the most effective management, particularly evidence from research on:

- **Chronicity**, i.e. Living with a chronic illness or long-term condition; chronic illnesses are the most significant health problem of the twenty-first century and some themes are common to all long-term conditions. There is a significant literature available on service configuration and the psychological impact of living with a chronic condition.
- **Wellbeing**: the psychology of resilience is important for those living with breathlessness: it is now clear that there are skills which all can learn to increase their 'mental capital.' Greater resilience can lead to more enjoyment of life, enhancing individuals' ability to take decisions and actions for themselves, in the face of difficulties. This is an area of emerging knowledge and is discussed in a later section of this chapter.
- **Communication skills**: breathlessness management often requires patients to change their lifestyle and learn new skills. People need to feel motivated to do this and helping them to achieve change will be more effective if the clinician has the right communication skills. Motivational interviewing techniques are particularly important.

- **Palliative care**; this speciality has researched and practised ways of helping patients facing life threatening illness by investigating and treating all symptoms, not only breathlessness, reducing anxiety, supporting carers and, when needed, giving excellent end of life care. Palliative care overlaps with supportive care which is simply those treatments that are not primarily directed at the illness but help an individual have the best physical and mental health possible. Many people with chronic intractable breathlessness are not immediately facing death. They need their clinicians to have the skills and attributes necessary for helping them to face a frightening reality in addition to clinical knowledge. These attributes include a disposition to empathise, show understanding, act with kindness and a motivation to manage symptoms as actively as investigating and treating disease.
- **Rehabilitation**: until the very end of life patients need to be treated as living sentient human beings capable of self efficacy, agency and the ability to change. Being able to look ahead with some sense of safety is important, even when very ill. This was demonstrated thoughout all the phases of evaluation of CBIS and is emerging from the evolving work on improving wellbeing.

  "At night, if the wrong things have popped into my head….worried….how long are you going to live….then you get breathless"

  – Female, Lung Ca, 53 year old.

For example, someone who is very ill but who can, even if temporarily, be helped to learn how to transfer from bed to chair unsupported, will have a greater chance of living at home until the end of their life.

Those with a longer prognosis have the opportunity to improve their health becoming fitter and more active if they are given the right sort of help.

- **Psychology, psychiatry and neuroscience**. People living with breathlessness, are helped by maintaining or improving their sense of self-efficacy to help overcome the accumulated assaults of illness. Depression, anxiety and other affective disorders are more common in those with chronic illness but can be treated, possibly prevented, greatly improving quality of life.

  It's getting your head into gear first….stop and think….relax and breathe…..It's not your last breath, it's not. If you just get your head into gear and just think, that's what they taught me anyway. It does work.
  – Male, Lung Ca, aged 58 participating in Booth et al. (2003)

- **Carers**; it is increasing recognised that the carers of those with chronic illness suffer increased ill-health, particularly ischaemic heart disease and depression. There is an increasing body of evidence on how to help carers. This is outlined in Chap. 9.

Evidence from all these areas forms the basis for specialist, multi-professional breathlessness services (often based in palliative care departments) for which there is increasing evidence. The breathlessness service approach will need to continue to evolve as new evidence emerges from all these areas, as it is a complex intervention. References for the evaluation of the Cambridge Breathlessness Intervention Service are given at the end of the chapter with review articles outlining the work of others.

> To continue to give your patients the best help it is important to keep looking for relevant work in these areas of research and to ensure that your service model is flexible and can evolve to meet changing needs in your geographical area.

First Steps in Assessment – Taking a History of the Patient's Breathlessness

This is discussed in detail in Chap. 2. It is very common to see guidance on how to take a detailed pain history, and a similar systematic approach to gathering information is just as important for effective breathlessness management. The history does not simply involve a litany of questions eliciting and encouraging one word answers, nor is it a rambling conversation (see Chap. 2). The structure of the interview comes from the patient; the clinician's focus is to discover information that will guide them to help the patient.

The first step towards giving good care for the breathless patients is to listen to their experience of the impact of breathlessness, to find out how it has affected that individual and those closest to them.

Breathlessness is an experience influenced by the higher thinking and feeling areas of the brain and by those more 'primitive' areas that respond almost reflexively or instantly to threat.

Breathlessness is an intrinsically threatening experience. It seems that humans are 'hard-wired' to feel anxious when experiencing breathlessness. The severity of that anxiety will be influenced by the higher centres (for e.g. by that individual's previous experience and/or interpretation of the symptom). A person can learn to reduce their feeling of breathlessness by using their minds (Table 12.1) (Gracely et al. 2007).

TABLE 12.1 Prompts for areas that need to be covered in assessment and reassessment of the breathless patient

History from the notes and other clinicians caring for that patient; obtain and read before any home visit or out-patients. Talk to other clinicians particularly GP or family physician or AHP or specialist nurses who know patients well.
History of breathlessness: onset, history, pattern, rate of progression, precipitating and alleviating factors, drugs taken to relieve, outcome of other treatments e.g. pulmonary rehabilitation, patients understanding and explanation for breathlessness . Are there crises? I.e. episodes of overwhelming breathlessness seemingly 'out of the blue'? Who does what at these times?
Family and support available; where? who does what? Who helps? Who hinders? Financial concerns, other agencies, charities which are involved.
Medical and clinical support; who does patient see as their regular clinician who is in overall charge? Who do they get on with best in this context? Do different clinicians give different types of support.
Action plan: decided with patient and carer
Advanced care planning? Now or later? (See Chap. 2)
Prescription? Opioids or other drugs needed now? If the patient is dying are the right drugs in the house?
Review? When and who? Where?
Carer? Any action?
Discharge back to? Who will carry on breathlessness interventions when you are no longer seeing? Do they have the right information from you to do this? Can patient be re-referred if necessary?
Liaison: with patients' clinical teams (they need to know what you have done and plan to do and how long you are seeing the patient) Record: the patient's caring teams will need a record of what you are doing but so will the patient. Small cards with prompts on, notices on the wall, letters written specifically for the patient can all be helpful here. Did you write a ritual for crises? The patient and carer will need a copy more than anyone.
Refer on: to pulmonary rehabilitation, to hospice services to another specialist. All this will need to be discussed with the patient and the patient's primary care physicians.

TABLE 12.1 (continued)

Information. Does the patient and carer have all the information they need, do they have information sheets, access to helpful website? Do the primary care team have the information they need to carry out supporting the patient's breathlessness treatment plan? Are there support agencies the patient is not using e.g. disease specific groups or charities?

Selecting an Intervention

Once you have a detailed history of the breathlessness and its impact you can begin to formulate, with the patient, a therapeutic plan to palliate the sensation and the difficulties it causes. The choice of the first intervention(s) to be selected for the individual will be governed by:

- Priority for patient: if someone has a particular short or long-term goal in mind, this will help prioritise the early interventions used. For example, if a father describes severe anxiety and breathlessness when in a crowded place, and wants to attend a son's school play, he may want to learn breathing retraining and anxiety reduction techniques first.
- Medical assessment: for example, if you feel there may be complicating thrombo-embolic disease, you will want to investigate this quickly (the sorts of investigations used being appropriate for that individual). You may need to make a referral to another specialist to ensure that treatment of the underlying, or another complicating condition is optimised.
- Patient's disposition and choices: some individuals will prefer a drug to manage anxiety rather than learning an anxiety reduction, strategy or vice versa. Whilst there are few drugs suitable for long-term use in anxiety, you might choose to use one initially to get improvement and build trust.

Always institute an intervention on the day that you first assess someone. There are a number of 'do no harm, likely to do good' pro-central, non-pharmacological interventions which increase self-efficacy and which be used in any one with breathlessness at any stage of the illness (see Box 12.1).

Box 12.1: 'Some examples of 'Do no harm, likely to do good' interventions'

- The hand-held fan, with education on how to use it
- Developing a 'ritual for crises' plan
- Breathing retraining
- Energy conservation and pacing
- Encouraging mental and physical activity and/or exercise
- Learning an anxiety reduction or relaxation technique
- Learning about wellbeing interventions
- Education on breathlessness
- Carer support and interventions

To institute *all* of these however, in detail, on the first occasion that you meet a breathless person would be too tiring and time-consuming for the patient. As you describe the rationale for a complex intervention, using a variety of approaches for managing breathlessness, you will touch on many, perhaps all of them, during discussion. You can use written information or the web to provide more ideas for the patient to consider in their own time, concentrating on the first visit on the intervention you think will have the biggest impact, most quickly.

It is important for the patient to start using one useful intervention that gives them back a measure of control from as early as possible, preferably at the first meeting.

Pro-central, Non-pharmacological Interventions

What are called, non-pharmacological interventions are the mainstay of the evidence-based, effective CBIS intervention. The word non-pharmacological is unsatisfactory as it does not convey either the type of intervention used, (and this term encompasses a multiplicity of treatments) nor the effectiveness of this group of treatments. Booth et al. (in preparation) and (Spathis et al. 2011) have proposed:

(i) a new term to replace the term 'non-pharmacological'
(ii) a classification of such interventions, at least until better ones can be found.

Pro-central is again a general term but it is a positive designation of these treatment strategies and postulates the way in which they modulate breathlessness. It has been proposed, with others, as a term to replace non-pharmacological and is not in general use.

Pro-central, non-pharmacological interventions can then be classified by the way they reduce the sensation of breathlessness (see Chaps. 1 and 2) by a primary effect on either:

Thinking: for example, cognitive behavioural therapy (CBT), education, wellbeing interventions, rituals for crises, carer support.

Breathing: for example, morphine and other opioids, the hand-held fan and other oro-nasal cooling methods, breathing retraining, draining pleural effusions.

Functioning; for example, exercise, pacing and energy conservation techniques, physical and metal activity.

It is clear that most pro-central, non-pharmacological interventions will affect more than one of these areas, but have their greatest impact in one. The terms are used also help clinicians understand a possible explanation for the effectiveness of the intervention they are using. This also helps the clinician teach these interventions to patients (and colleagues) in an informed way.

Active informed listening by a clinicians interested in breathlessness is a pro-central intervention in itself; this was clearly demonstrated in the data from the CBIS evaluation over ten years.

Summary of 'the Complex Intervention, Breathlessness Service' Approach

The majority of patients that many breathlessness services see have advanced COPD but an increasing proportion are reaching out to see those with lung cancer, interstitial lung disease (ILD) or heart failure, which all have a much shorter prognosis. The treatment strategy for what can be called chronic breathlessness (lasting many months or years) and for rapidly-progressive breathlessness (weeks to months) are similar but have a different emphasis. **The principles are outlined in Table** 12.2. End of life care is different, and has been discussed in Chap. 11.

TABLE 12.2 Some key differences in the approaches to managing chronic and rapidly progressive breathlessness

Chronic breathlessness lasting years	Rapidly progressive or severe breathlessness with a prognosis of weeks to months
Drug therapy less favoured for palliation dyspnoea	More emphasis on drug therapy for palliation of dyspnoea
Benzodiazepines rarely used (risk of dependency/difficulty withdrawing)	Benzodiazepines used as necessary to help anxiety
Emphasis on engaging patients with life outside medical sphere (e.g. sports or activities to be continued in longer term to promote exercise and mental and physical fitness) as well as appropriate services supporting treatment of breathlessness e.g. pulmonary rehabilitation	Emphasis on engaging patients with other services that help end of life care and offer extra support to carers e.g. community nurse, hospice services.

Table 12.2 (continued)

Chronic breathlessness lasting years	**Rapidly progressive or severe breathlessness with a prognosis of weeks to months**
Emphasis on increasing physical activity continuously. Support of current, & development of new, social relationships	Emphasis on activity both physical and mental that fits with patient's physical condition at that moment
Emphasis on prevention of longer term morbidity e.g. from corticosteroids, from smoking, from inactivity, from cardiac complications of COPD, from poor nutrition, from systemic inflammation	Emphasis on minimising drug burden reducing need to change 'habits of lifetime.' Review particularly those drugs which are aimed at prevention of longer morbidity and have uncertain role for that individual in last days, weeks or months of life.
Emphasis on helping carers get support outside medical systems and to look after their own health	Emphasis on clinical services that can help the carer survive period of patient's rapid decline and death, helping them into life outside clinical services afterwards e.g. hospice services
Emphasis on healthy nutrition to minimise chances of obesity, diabetes mellitus, heart disease. Possible role for interventions that may reduce inflammation e.g. fish oils.	Emphasis on enjoying whatever food is palatable and adjusting diet to minimise symptoms for example if cancer complicated by partial bowel obstruction eating a low fibre diet.
Emphasis on using wellbeing strategies to enhance resilience (See section below)	Concentrating on those approaches which already work for the patient, even if adopted in the longer term would not be the currently evidence-based approach. Longer-term wellbeing interventions can be used for carers.

Deciding When Drug Therapy is Needed for Palliation of Breathlessness

The question of drug therapy (including oxygen) for breathlessness was discussed in detail in Chaps. 3 and 10. The decision to prescribe or not is again mentioned here as it is important in designing an overall approach to the symptoms.

It is especially important to consider whether pharmacological treatment is appropriate in patients with a prognosis of years rather than months or weeks.

There are few drugs available to palliate breathlessness which have a significant evidence base. This will change in the future but currently we have only opioids for direct palliation (which have been tested in randomised controlled trials), plus mirtazapine and benzodiazepines which may have a dual action and a minimal evidence base.

Opioids give at best a 20 % improvement in breathlessness – the range quoted is 8–20 %. They can have adverse effects, although these can be treated with varying degrees of success, depending on the individual. They have not been tested in longer term trials; the evidence available has tested opioids over months at maximum and there was significant attrition of patients from the trials. Most of the patients in these trials had non-malignant breathlessness mostly from COPD.

In a patient reaching the end of life, which includes all those breathless at rest or on very minimal exertion, opioids should be, an early choice to help palliate the symptom.

In mobile patients it is better to palliate using a predominantly non-pharmacological approach, with support and explaining why a procentral, non-drug approach is preferable, where possible.

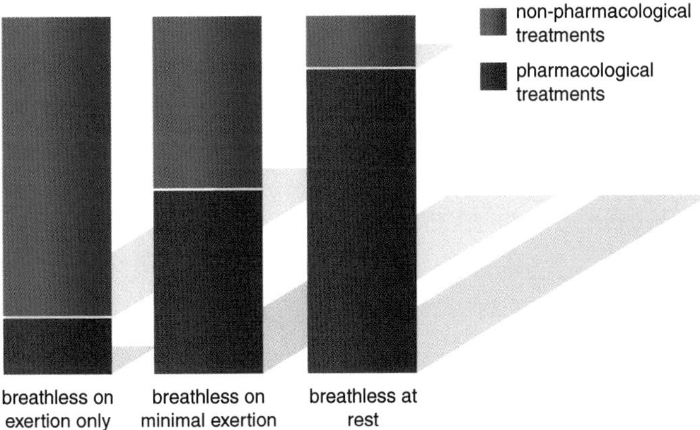

FIGURE 12.1 Graph to show relative contributions of non-pharmacological and pharmacological treatments for breathlessness at different stages of an illness. *First bar*: breathless on exertion only. *Second bar*: breathless on minimal exertion. *Third bar*: breathless at rest. *Blue* = non-pharmacological treatments. *Red* = pharmacological treatments

Andrew Wilcock summarised the balance of non-pharmacological to pharmacological approaches well in his graph reproduced in (Fig. 12.1).

A complex non-pharmacological approach needs the clinician to do more work initially but if successful can bring about longer-term change which can improve the patient's general health. Complex interventions work in multiple ways to enhance care, and can potentially reduce the patient's need for support from health services. Clinicians themselves may need extra training to learn, for example, motivational interviewing and how to build the patient's confidence in carrying out physical activities.

Most non-pharmacological interventions work in several ways; nearly all increase the patient's sense of self-efficacy and need some education from the clinician to be most effective. An example is given in Box 12.2

> Box 12.2
> "Considering the hand held fan, there is evidence that if it is simply handed to patients without explanation ('thinking') of how it affects afferent signals to the respiratory centre, ('breathing') how it is best employed in shortening recovery time after exercise ('functioning'), encouragement to have it always to hand ('thinking'), how the carer may be involved by giving it to the patient when breathless ('thinking'), its impact will be lessened "(Booth 2013a, b).

There are reasons for caution with the use of drugs for long-term palliation including:

- The impact and development of adverse effects have not been assessed in the long-term (i.e. years) for opioids, to date, opioids have mainly been used for patients entering the last months or weeks of life.
- There are questions being asked about the possible adverse impact of opioids on breathing patterns and nocturnal oxygenation.
- Drugs palliating breathlessness work both in the CNS and, where used topically, peripherally in the lungs. Most non-pharmacological agents have several modes of action (see below). An exception is mirtazapine which, should it prove to be more effective than usual care for breathlessness, would be affecting mood and breathlessness. There are data on adverse effects in longer term use and it seems to be safe.

Most non-pharmacological (pro-central) techniques require the person to undergo a training, to learn new skills. The clinician needs to have coaching skills, motivating and supporting the patient to persist with new techniques which may initially be difficult to learn.

The non-pharmacological interventions which do not require the patient to learn new skills are those needed by the physician throughout the disease course, but particularly as the end of life approaches.

> Kind, empathetic, listening on the part of the clinician, giving support, encouragement and education, an understanding of what will make the patient and family's life easier, i.e. problem solving and a disposition to act quickly, without erecting bureaucratic barriers, to help patient and family

Other Symptoms: Making a Full Assessment of the Breathless Patient

A palliative care assessment involves an understanding of the entirety of the patient's concerns – physical, psychological, social and spiritual and acting on those most important to that person first. It is clear that any separation of interventions, any attempt to define them as affecting one component of a distressing symptom or another is artificial. It is necessary to break down complex management regimens into comprehensible streams for the purposes of learning and teaching.

It is important, whatever your clinical background, to ensure that you have:

- Enquired about all symptoms, some other symptoms are particularly commonly found with breathlessness e.g. fatigue, cough and sputum retention.
- Found out from the patient which symptom(s) the patient wants treated most urgently, sometimes patients with cancer want their pain treated first; patients with ILD may want their cough treated first.
- Found out how the patient understands or explains the causes of their breathlessness – you may find that the patient (or carer) has some misconceptions about the symptom or its treatment. Common ones include (i)

getting breathless should be avoided (this leads to deconditioning and worsening of breathlessness), or (ii) continuous rest is the best treatment, another belief that has the same harmful consequences.

A carer of one patient was discouraging him from exercise because she thought her relative's heart was damaged by the illness. A letter from the consultant caring for that patient clarifying in writing that this was not so, gave the necessary reassurance and contributed to a great increase in that patient's fitness and consequently, quality of life.

General Treatment Strategies for People with Chronic Conditions

The specific treatments for breathlessness have been outlined earlier in this book but there are others which will help anyone living with a chronic condition. Some of these cross with specific management strategies for breathlessness.

All people with chronic illnesses need to:

- Exercise or at least be as active as possible
- Maintain and develop new social relationships.
- Eat in a way that builds rather than lessens health.
- Enhance their sense of resilience and wellbeing.
- Maintain or improve their sense of self-efficacy i.e. their sense of being able to influence the outcome of events that overtake them.
- Keep mentally active

The science of wellbeing, associated with maintaining or improving 'personal mental capital' (contributing to resilience) throughout life is particularly important in those with a chronic illness as:

(i) depression worsens medical outcomes
(ii) people with chronic illness have more physical difficulties and mental disappointments than those who are healthy, predisposing to anxiety and depression

(iii) those with a sense of wellbeing are more likely to carry out actions that will benefit them and those around them.

The relevant evidence suggests that a sense of wellbeing comprises:

1. a sense of engagement with the world around us
2. a sense of being involved with something larger of more significant than ourselves as individuals
3. enjoying pleasurable activities

There has been considerable progress in this area in the past five years and it is important to consider this aspect of care when helping patients to manage their illness and supporting those closest to them.

The Foresight programme (HMG Office for Science) brought together neuroscientists, psychologists, and psychiatrists and others with expertise in every stage of life, to examine the evidence in this area. As well as several helpful reports and CDs, the 'new economics foundation' (a think tank) produced some postcards which encapsulate the evidence. They are 'prompts to actions' that will build resilience, in an attractive and comprehensible form. These may be freely used in clinical practice, with appropriate acknowledgement.

Five ways to wellbeing

Foresight's Mental Capital and Wellbeing Project has drawn on state-of-the-art research from across the world to consider how to improve everyone's mental capital and mental wellbeing through life.

Evidence suggests that a small improvement in wellbeing can help to decrease some mental health problems and also help people to flourish.

The Project commissioned the centre for well-being at **nef** (the new economics foundation) to develop 'five ways to wellbeing': a set of evidence-based actions to improve personal wellbeing.

Five ways
to wellbeing

Be active...

Go for a walk or run. Step outside. Cycle. Play a game. Garden. Dance. Exercising makes you feel good. Most importantly, discover a physical activity you enjoy and one that suits your level of mobility and fitness.

Five ways
to wellbeing

Connect...

Connect with the people around you. With family, friends, colleagues and neighbours. At home, work, school or in your local community. Think of these as the cornerstones of your life and invest time in developing them. Building these connections will support and enrich you every day.

Five ways
to wellbeing

Give…

Do something nice for a friend, or a stranger. Thank someone. Smile. Volunteer your time. Join a community group. Look out, as well as in. Seeing yourself, and your happiness, linked to the wider community can be incredibly rewarding and creates connections with the people around you.

Five ways
to wellbeing

Keep learning…

Try something new. Rediscover an old interest. Sign up for that course. Take on a different responsibility at work. Fix a bike. Learn to play an instrument or how to cook your favourite food. Set a challenge you will enjoy achieving. Learning new things will make you more confident as well as being fun.

Five ways
to wellbeing

Take notice...

Be curious. Catch sight of the beautiful. Remark on the unusual. Notice the changing seasons. Savour the moment, whether you are walking to work, eating lunch or talking to friends. Be aware of the world around you and what you are feeling. Reflecting on your experiences will help you appreciate what matters to you.

The postcards are particularly valuable because the patient (or other user) decides how to implement the actions that will help build their health. Like the fan, it will be important to explain the science behind the 'prompts' rather than simply just handing them out.

'**There is no evidence**.'

Most people with chronic illness will seek advice on living with the condition from the internet, the press social media, patient support groups, and friends with the same or other chronic condition, relatives, and self-help books. They will often use complementary therapists. The terms 'alternative' or 'complementary' when used to refer to therapists or treatments are broad and encompass some helpful individuals and approaches and some which are both expensive and frankly dangerous.

The reasons that people look outside their clinical team for help with managing their condition are many but may include:

- they do not get the empathy and understanding they need about their predicament from their clinical team

- they want to see if there is anything else that can be done to cure or at least improve their condition or reduce their suffering and sense of isolation
- they fear that doctors (and other health professionals) will only recommend 'conventional' or 'allopathic' treatments regardless of whether other strategies may help
- they are dying, there is no further allopathic treatment to prolong life and they want (like the great majority) to live as long as they possibly can
- they have heard about someone who has their condition who has been cured or lived longer with a specific treatment/diet/complementary therapy
- they need psychological support and do not get it from their clinical team
- they want to do something for themselves to improve their condition or general health
- they suffer with anxiety and want to find something that will help with that.
- they have physical symptoms for which there appear to be no further helpful strategies

Some of the most common complementary therapies used are dietary (e.g. the use of an exclusive diet and/or the use of supplements). There are many other therapies varying from transcendental meditation to Reiki, to massage, reflexology, self-hypnosis, aromatherapy, crystal therapy and so on.

It is some patients' experience that when they tell their clinicians about their use of an alternative therapy they experience a response that feels dismissive and possibly contemptuous. Very often the clinician will say 'There is no evidence for that.'

This is unhelpful in many ways:

- the patient may feel dismissed and belittled and then angry and less likely to listen to any real concerns the clinician may have about the alternative treatment
- the patient will not in the future, discuss any complementary therapies they are trying, this could be dangerous either because the therapy is potentially harmful or because it contains active ingredients that could interact with standard treatments

There are different reasons why potential interventions do not have research to support them. It may be that there is no evidence because it has not been looked for or it may be there is no evidence because good research has been done and the intervention has no evidence to support its use. It may be because there is no reason to think that it will help or that it is likely to be dangerous.

These reasons (and there are others) are markedly different.

What you cannot do.

> As a clinician you cannot recommend treatments or support the use of therapies that are outside your scope of knowledge or for which there is no evidence-base, or, of course, for which there is evidence of harm. Remember, however, that many allopathic treatments in current use are based upon best practice, rather than Grade evidence, particularly in palliative care.

Many complementary treatments are really complex interventions where the context of care, the rituals around treatment and the listening by the therapist of the patient probably play a part in any therapeutic effect.

Many complex interventions have not been investigated because

1. they are not pharmaceutical and therefore the expensive investigation necessary is not supported by drug companies
2. they are complicated and difficult to investigate e.g. dietary interventions, e.g. exercise e.g. meditation
3. suitable outcome measures have not been designed to measure the impact of that intervention

An intervention may not be useless, just not investigated rigorously yet.

What you can do:

- listen attentively to the reasons and the rationale the patient has for using that intervention (you may identify a deficiency in your own service).

- Give a considered opinion on it, (you may need to look something up or take advice from colleagues). Say that you need to understand more about it to the patient, don't support or discourage something you know nothing about unless it sounds as if it is actively or potentially dangerous (e.g. an unknown supplement or a very high dose of a standard supplement like vitamin A). Find out from the patient about any active constituents of something they are taking and ask them to stop taking it until you can find out more about it. Knowing the constituents enables you immediately to rule out harmful interventions e.g. silver salts.
- If you think it is actually dangerous or likely to interfere with a treatment you using, explain and advise strongly about future use.
- If the treatment is doing no harm and may do good (perhaps through an as yet unexplained phenomenon, often described by the term 'placebo effect') explain this and be supportive of it, making it clear that it will not cure, outlining any other limitations on it.
- Express concern if you think the patients is spending too much money and being encouraged to have high expectations of the results of the intervention.
- Extreme diets can be dangerous but so can no advice or dismissive advice about diets too.
- If the patient wants to try a complementary therapy, it may be that it is safely offered at low cost by a local hospice or self-help group e.g. Maggie centre.
- Remember that some treatments are now actively promoted that were once dismissed as 'alternative' e.g. vitamin D, exercise, meditation, fish oils.
- With dietary supplements, sometimes called nutraceuticals, the dose is important. For example, many people do not realise that Vitamin A is dangerous in too high a dose.
- Remember that some accepted mainstream clinical interventions employ dietary manipulation or use supplementation e.g. in renal disease, e.g. reducing dietary sodium and increasing dietary potassium in hypertension, e.g. magnesium in pre-eclampsia

Use Your Common Sense

(i) you may feel you know nothing about dietary interventions but if your patient is existing on burgers, chips, fizzy drinks, doughnuts and other high fat, trans fat and high sugar foods they are eating an unhealthy diet and simply because they like it, it is not to be encouraged, except at the end of life (when people rarely want to eat that sort of food). They need advice from a qualified dietician.

(ii) If the intervention will not harm, even if you are sceptical, e.g. Reiki, provided that patient is not spending too much money or investing too much hope in it, why oppose or belittle it? Your patient will be unlikely to tell you about other attempts to use complementary therapies if you do. That does not mean you encourage it because of a possible anti-disease effect.

Reviewing the Evidence

You may have to look outside your specialist area to find the evidence you need and it may be imperfect but an intervention without RCT or a systematic review may be worth trying if

1. there is a rationale behind it
2. there is some case report evidence plus a rationale
3. the patient is desperate or there is little other treatment available and the treatment can do no harm
4. it promotes something else that is healthy e.g. self efficacy and/or exercise

Example – The Hand-Held Fan

Some authorities will say that the fan has little evidence to back up its use in breathlessness but:

1. it cannot do harm
2. its use is clearly palliative not curative

3. there has long been a physiological rationale and some small studies suggesting why it might work
4. it promotes self efficacy
5. there is now mass of qualitative data and one small RCT from patients supporting its use
6. it is cheap
7. it has no adverse effects

In contrast, to take a fabricated example, radiotherapy for toothache

1. is potentially dangerous
2. is very expensive using many precious health service resources
3. it promotes passivity
4. has no rationale to suggest it might be useful
5. it has very serious side effects

In evaluating complementary therapy and interventions that you can potentially offer in your own service, you must take a scientific approach allied with a broad outlook which focuses on the patient's goals and a wider interpretation of health.

Breathlessness Services

There is now increasing evidence that breathlessness services can increase the quality of care given to patients with this distressing symptom.

The abstract of RCT of the CBIS comparing 'usual care' against 'CBIS and usual care' in patients with cancer, published in 2012 (full paper under review), demonstrated that for patients with breathless of any aetiology the CBIS significantly reduced 'distress due to breathlessness' and 94 % of people felt that they had been helped a lot (68 %) or somewhat (24 %) by the service (Farquhar et al. 2011). Patients and carers were able to name *identifiable, specific and teachable* interventions that had helped including the hand-held fan, breathing retraining, support for carers, energy conservation and pacing that had helped reduced the impact of the symptom. Health care costs were lower in patients using the service.

Other breathlessness services related to CBIS have been set up at King's college London, in Halifax Nova Scotia and there is one developing in Munich (Booth et al. 2011a, b). There are also a number of breathlessness clinics at hospices in the UK and throughout the world (Booth et al. 2011c).

The advantage of a service is that there is a uniformity of the standard of care given to breathless patients. It also creates a specialist fount of knowledge within a locality which can support other clinicians working with breathless patients by giving advice and seeing specific patients.

Some different models are outlined in Table 12.3

Principles of Setting Up a Breathlessness Service

If you want to set up breathlessness service and you have no extra funding think about the following:

- What sort of clinicians do I have available to work with breathless patients?
- What other resources exist in my area? For example, hospice day centre or pulmonary rehabilitation. You may able to start doing some work through these existing channels
- What sorts of patients with breathlessness are most common in my area? Perhaps for you patients with asbestosis or cystic fibrosis or lung cancer have the greatest need and least help, start working with these patients first and gain the support of the specialists in that team.
- Demonstrate need, perhaps by a survey or by calculating the number in each disease group and working out how many have advanced disease and therefore are likely to be breathless
- Is there a charity (local or national) that could support some extra clinician time for a defined period, during which you would work to demonstrate improvement in outcomes.

If you do start a service ensure you have some outcome measures – use those which would have most impact in your vicinity, usually a mixture of improved patient outcomes and

TABLE 12.3 Examples of different service models for breathless patients

Name of service	BIS	BSS	ICON	Inspired	Advanced resp care MDTS
Composition	1.0 wte spec OT, 0.4 wte consultant physician, 1.0 wte spec physio, 0.6 wte admin. Access to psychologist	1.0 wte physio, 0.1 wte consultants in resp med & pall care, nurse, social worker	1.0 wte OT, 0.5 physio, 0.2 wte consultant physician	1.0 respiratory therapist and consultant physician	Variable but usually weekly or monthly meeting of services e.g., pall care and resp med (community, hospital and hospice services)
Based in	Hospital pall care service	Hospital pall care service	hospice	Hospital resp med dept	Variable, often rotate site of meeting
Operates in	Community, hospital wards & clinics (less common)	Community, out patients	Community & hospice	Community & hospital	Communication on patients in all settings
Distinctive feature	Sees most patients at home, transition team for patients on ward.	Resp med & social work involvement	Enables patients to get to hospice using taxis & rolling programme of interventions ‘drop in as needed.’	Covers huge geographical area, unusual mix in resp med	Meeting of acute, community & hospice personnel

Booth et al. 2011a–c

more effective health care expenditure such as reduced hospital admissions with improved care at home.

Do some 'before' and 'after' measurements to demonstrate improved patient outcomes plus reduced spend. Of course, reduced spend and reduced quality of care for patients is a bad outcome. You need both increased quality with reduced cost, possibly by reducing spend elsewhere in the health system.

Details of service design can be found in 'The BIS manual' and there is now excellent evidence from at least two specialist breathlessness services that demonstrate effectiveness of this approach.

Who to Call and When

One of the most unhelpful actions that a service can take when working with patients in the community is to fail to make it clear who they can call when they need help.

All too often the unhelpful phrase, 'Call us if there is a problem' is used at the end of a visit.

Patients with advanced chronic disease already have multiple problems and need advice on

- **When** they should call for help i.e. what signs will show that they need help, reassuring them it is right to call for help when it is needed even at the weekend or in the middle of the night
- **Where to call**; patients and families need information about numbers for services and when these are available. It is particularly important, even if everything looks stable when you see someone on a Friday, to clarify which numbers patients and families should use if they need help over the weekend.
- **Who to call**: patients and families need to know who they should call first. This may be different (although this is not ideal) for different situations or times of day. The most important thing is that patients have a number to ring where someone will respond; again if a separate number is needed for 'out of hours' it is important to give it.

- **What numbers to use**; and what to do if there is no response
- **How**; services may use landlines or mobiles and there may even email contact for some resources.

What can you do in Your Setting to Help Breathless Patients?

Health services all over the world are trying to spend less or at least stabilise how much is spent on health care. Setting up a new service in your area may not be possible or may take some time.

You can start today to help breathless patients by first:

(i) Taking steps to go out and identify people with this symptom, they are often 'hidden' or 'silent.'
(ii) applying best current practice (see below)
(iii) educating and supporting other clinicians to do the same

Summary of Current Best Practice in Managing Breathlessness (Johnson and Booth 2010, Ahmedzai et al. 2012)

(i) assessing the patient by **active listening** and hearing about their goals and priorities, including the presence of other symptoms which may be exacerbating the breathlessness
(ii) a personal exercise programme reversing **deconditioning**, of a sort that will be continued in the longer run, not only as 'exercise' but also as part of an enjoyable life. Finding a sport or physical activity that the individual enjoys is important, rather than trying to prescribe a joyless exercise programme to be continued, without clinical support, indefinitely. In the less well patient, activity is important, both physical and mental.
(iii) **modifying the central perception** of dyspnoea e.g. education, psychological approaches, drugs in those who are less mobile or more distressed (opioids first line)
(iv) education about **pacing** and **energy conservation**
(v) **breathing retraining**, including use of the fan

(vi) **enhancing wellbeing** e.g. building resilience using positive psychological interventions and possibly meditative approaches such as mindfulness-based stress reduction (MBSR)
(vii) treating **depression**
(viii) **carer support and education**
(ix) treating **any other symptom** actively; fatigue and cough are very common in breathless patients

Disseminating Your Practice

You must ensure that when you have seen a patient everyone else involved in that patient's care knows what you have done, and why, your plans for future care for that patient and what will be needed when you discharge them from your care (if you are not in primary care). Other clinicians who do not know about breathlessness need help finding out the information they need to help that patient. They may not know that exercise is helpful; they may not know that the hospices can help a patient with non-malignant disease; they may not know how badly the carer is faring (patient and carers may have different GPs.)

Communicating is vital and needs to be continued by you throughout the period of time you are seeing the patient. A phone call at some stage to other clinicians is often very helpful.

Linda is 17 years and has been treated for a childhood cancer. Although cured she is disabled by breathlessness as the high dose chemotherapy necessary had damaged her lungs. She is breathless on the slightest exertion. She is ambitious and wants to catch up with her academic work and go to university. Her loving parents have been terribly frightened by her disease and restrict her activity. She feels trapped as she needs their help to do anything and lives at home. Her mother always comes to clinic with her. The Breathlessness service sees her at home. Linda particularly valued the exercise and breathing retraining advice she was given. She had discussed various interests that she could take up with the OT and decided to look at photography which had both intellectual and physical aspects to recommend it. It also did not frighten her mother, who had been reassured after talking through exercise training with the physiotherapist and understood its possible value for Linda, she had not understood that being breathless after exertion could be a positive outcome.

Linda's photography improved, she decided to take it as an 'A' level option and joined a photography club. She felt able to join club outings and the club member were very willing to make it possible for her to come out with them. Linda won a photography prize and went to college to take it further. It offered a possible way of earning a living and contributed greatly to an increased sense of hope and self esteem. Linda gradually became much fitter, she took up golf at the local pay and play after some lessons. The drugs she needed for her lung condition could be decreased. Gradually and happily she and her parents readjusted their relationship and Linda moved out to complete her MA and then take up part time employment.

Excellent management of breathlessness should be possible for all patients and their families: clinicians of any training can at least initiate it and then work with colleagues with specialist skills and experience to improve their care further. The first step is to listen to the patient, recognising the impact of the symptom on that individual's life and the consequent effects on those around them. This is the remit of all clinicians. Next some simple evidence-based treatments can be started, some of which are appropriate for patients with any chronic condition. Then discussion with and possibly referral to colleagues may be needed for the individual to get the best care possible. Breathlessness can be helped if clinicians familiarise themselves with the latest evidence in this area and have the determination to apply it. To sum up by using Eleanor Roosevelt's sentiment, if not her exact words,

> Do what you can, where you are with what you have got.

Key Points

- Intractable breathlessness should always have a diagnosed cause and optimisation of the treatment of the underlying condition should have been completed.
- Breathlessness can be improved by use of a complex intervention which is designed around the patient's goals and priorities and based on the available evidence
- Breathlessness services which take a rehabilitative approach can be helpful in improving the care of breathless patients.
- Carers need help too.
- It is helpful to start an intervention at the time of assessment.
- Help those living with breathlessness (patients and carers) to improve their mental resilience.

References

Ahmedzai S, Currow D, Baldwin D. Supportive care in respiratory disease. 2nd ed. Oxford: OUP; 2012.

Booth S, Silvester S, Todd CJ. Breathlessness in cancer and chronic obstructive pulmonary disease: using a qualitative approach to describe the experience of patients and carers. Palliat Support Care. 2003;1:337–44.

Booth S, Bausewein C, Rocker G. New models of care for advanced lung disease. Prog Palliat Care. 2011a;19(5):254–63.

Booth S, Moffat C, Burkin J, Galbraith S, Bausewein C. Non pharmacological interventions for breathlessness. Curr Opin Support Palliat Care. 2011b;5(2):77–86.

Booth S, Moffat C, Farquhar M, Higginson IJ, Burkin J. Developing a breathlessness intervention service for patients with palliative and supportive care needs, irrespective of diagnosis. J Palliat Care. 2011c;27(1):28–36.

Booth S. The wellbeing diary. Cambridge: Addenbrookes Palliative Care Service and the Fitzwilliam Museum; Dandelion Clock, 2013a.

Booth S. Science supporting the art of medicine; improving the management of breathlessness. Palliat Med. 2013b;27(6):483–5.

Farquhar M, Prevost AT, McCrone P, Higginson IJ, Gray J, Brafman-Kennedy B, Booth S. Study protocol: phase III single-blinded fast-track pragmatic randomised controlled trial of a complex intervention for breathlessness in advanced disease. Trials. 2011;12:130.

Gracely RH, Undem BJ and Banzett RB. Cough, pain and dyspnoea: similarities and differences. Pulm Pharmacol Ther. 2007;20(4):433–437.

Johnson MJ, Booth S. Palliative and end of life care for patients with chronic heart failure and chronic lung disease. Clin Med. 2010;10(3):1–4.

Spathis A, Davies HE, Booth S. Respiratory disease; from advanced disease to bereavement. Oxford: OUP; 2011.

Further Reading

Booth S, Farquhar M, Gysels M, Bausewein C, Higginson I. The impact of a breathlessness intervention service (BIS) on the lives of patients with intractable dyspnoea: a qualitative phase 1 study. Palliat Support Care. 2006;4:287–93.

Foresight Mental Capital and Wellbeing Project. Final project report – executive summary. London: The Government Office for Science; 2008.

Wellbeing Postcards reproduced with permission of the Government Office for Science and the nef (new economics foundation), London.

Index

S. Booth et al., *Managing Breathlessness in Clinical Practice*,
DOI 10.1007/978-1-4471-4754-1_1,

N

O

P

Printed in Great Britain
by Amazon.co.uk, Ltd.,
Marston Gate.